Nutrition and Cancer
From Epidemiology to Biology

Editors

Pier Paolo Claudio & Richard M. Niles

Joan C. Edwards School of Medicine
Marshall University
Nutrition and Cancer Center
Translational Research Genomic Institute
Department of Biochemistry and Microbiology
Huntington, WV, 25705
USA

eBooks End User License Agreement

CONTENTS

CHAPTERS

FOREWORD

In writing this forward, I was reminded by the common phrase, "you are what you eat", which implies that to remain healthy one must eat healthy foods. Scientists and health professionals have long recognized the benefits of eating healthy and in selecting foods that contain specific disease preventing nutrients and micronutrients. It is now well established that nutrients in the diet prevent or retard several processes associated with cancer; however, they also can contribute to cancer risk and progression. Non-nutritive, phytochemicals present in plants are powerful antineoplastic agents on their own and can enhance the response of patients to cancer therapies or prevent cancer reoccurrence, areas that are often under appreciated by medical practitioners.

While the information on nutrition and cancer is voluminous, the scientific data have not always lead to unambiguous recommendations regarding the role of nutrition in cancer prevention and progression. Because cancer is a collection of over 100 different diseases, various types of cancer and even cancers of the same type can express differential sensitivity to nutrients and phytochemicals making it difficult to discern their beneficial or detrimental effects. The mechanisms by which nutrients and phytochemicals modulate the assorted steps involved in the cancer process are themselves multifactorial and eclectic. Such is the nature of the topics in this book.

The book includes chapters on the current state of knowledge of noteworthy plant phytochemicals such as resveratrol found in high amounts in red wine, berries, and nuts, catechins found in green tea, and capsaicin present in chili peppers. It also includes timely information on emerging areas such as the role and epigenetic mechanisms of omega 3 fatty acids present in fatty fish and nuts, which are associated with cancer prevention and therapy. Oxidative stress is generally thought to promote cancer progression, and this subject is very effectively integrated into the book *via* the chapters discussing the relationship between heme iron from red meat, oxidative stress, and breast cancer, the receptor independent effects of retinoids related to changes in cellular oxidative state, and lastly the complexity associated with the antioxidant mechanisms of various phytochemicals including, but not limited to, resveratrol and those found in green tea.

While we as individuals cannot modify our genetic makeup and may have little control over the multitude of carcinogens in our environment, we have the power to make healthy diet-based choices that can significantly modify cancer risk and progression. The authors have structured this book not only to review the epidemiological studies that support the roles of selected nutrients/phytochemicals in cancer control, but also they review the cellular and molecular pathways involved in their action as well as the clinical data related to their efficacy in cancer treatment. Consequently, this book has wide appeal not only to researchers in the nutrition and cancer field, but also to oncology practitioners, dieticians, as well as cancer survivors, who are interested learning how healthy dietary choices can enhance their quality of life.

Gary G. Meadows,
Washington State University
Pullman, Washington
USA

PREFACE

Cancer is one of the leading causes of death in America. It is estimated that 42% of Americans living today may develop cancer in their lifetime. In 1971, President Nixon declared the new, aggressive "War on Cancer." In spite of these efforts, cancer death rates continue to climb. Unfortunately, this is in part due to the fact that chemotherapy and radiation have not provided the cure for cancer that was once promised. Furthermore, changes in lifestyle and dietary habits occurred, as we become a more industrialized civilization. The convenience of readily available high fat processed foods has resulted in individuals not always acquiring all the dietary components needed for proper wellbeing.

Various estimates suggest that between 30-40% of all human cancers are related to dietary patterns. Strong epidemiological evidence from population and twin studies point to dietary constituents that either contribute or protect against the development of various forms of cancer. Nutrition is a low cost, non-toxic therapy that can help to prevent or significantly delay the onset of certain cancers. Dietary constituents or supplements may also interact either in a positive or negative fashion with therapeutics agents used to treat patients with cancer.

The scientific community and the public are becoming increasingly aware of the cancer-preventive potential of a diet low in saturated fat/processed foods and high in whole grains, fruits and vegetables. Research on nutrition and effects upon cancer progression and development has become a leading topic among cancer researchers. This book is a timely collection of chapters based on research conducted by leading experts in the field of nutrition and cancer.

Research in nutrition and cancer prevention has significantly advanced our understanding of the mechanistic actions of various food components in cancer prevention. What we eat on a daily basis has a very powerful effect on our health and quality of life. By avoiding factors that increase the risk of certain cancer and including foods that protect us against this disease, we can, to a certain extent, control our own risk. Dietary components affect multiple cellular pathways and moderately inhibit or stimulate enzymes in these pathways. These actions may account for the nontoxic effects of phytochemicals and the relative lack of resistance that cancers develop to these compounds. New research suggests that multiple components of food substances have greater biologic activity than any one isolated component. This finding supports the pleiotropic action of diet and provides a potential explanation for why cancer cells do not quickly develop resistance.

This book reviews some traditional and relatively new areas of nutrition and cancer. Each chapter is written from an interdisciplinary viewpoint that combines epidemiological data with molecular biology research and where available clinical trial data. This book targets not only cancer researchers and clinicians, but also those who are interested in understanding how nutritional habits can impact our quality of life.

Pier Paolo Claudio & Richard M. Niles
Joan C. Edwards School of Medicine
Marshall University
Nutrition and Cancer Center
Translational Research Genomic Institute
Department of Biochemistry and Microbiology
Huntington, WV, 25705
USA

List of Contributors

Kathleen C. Brown

Department of Pharmacology, Physiology and Toxicology
Marshall University, Huntington, WV, 25755, USA

Pier Paolo Claudio

Department of Biochemistry and Microbiology
Marshall University, Huntington, WV, 25755, USA

Piyali Dasgupta

Department of Pharmacology, Physiology and Toxicology
Marshall University, Huntington, WV, 25755, USA

Aaron M. Dom

Department of Pharmacology, Physiology and Toxicology
Marshall University, Huntington, WV, 25755, USA

Richard D. Egleton

Department of Pharmacology, Physiology and Toxicology
Marshall University, Huntington, WV, 25755, USA

Elaine Hardman

Department of Biochemistry and Microbiology
Marshall University, Huntington, WV, 25755, USA

Kinsley Kelley Kiningham

Department of Pharmaceutical Sciences
Belmont University School of Pharmacy, Nashville, TN, 37212, USA

Jamie K. Lau

Department of Pharmacology, Physiology and Toxicology
Marshall University, Huntington, WV, 25755, USA

Richard M. Niles

Department of Biochemistry and Microbiology
Marshall University, Huntington, WV, 25755, USA

Gary Rankin

Department of Pharmacology, Physiology and Toxicology
Marshall University, Huntington, WV, 25755, USA

Nalini Santanam

Department of Pharmacology, Physiology and Toxicology
Marshall University, Huntington, WV, 25755, USA

Anne Silvis

Department of Pharmacology, Physiology and Toxicology
Marshall University, Huntington, WV, 25755, USA

Vincent Sollars

Department of Biochemistry and Microbiology
Marshall University, Huntington, WV, 25755, USA

Monica Valentovic

Department of Pharmacology, Physiology and Toxicology
Marshall University, Huntington, WV, 25755, USA

John Wilkinson IV

Department of Anatomy and Pathology
Marshall University, Huntington, WV, 25755, USA

Mary Allison Wolf

Department of Biochemistry and Microbiology
Marshall University, Huntington, WV, 25755, USA

Keywords List

13-cis RA, isotretinoin

All-trans Retinoic Acid

Angiogenesis

Apoptosis

Arachidonic Acid

Autophagy

Benzyl Isothiocyanate

Breast Cancer

Broccoli

Brussels Sprouts

Cabbage

Caffeine

Camellia sinensis

Cancer

Cancer Stem Cells

Capsaicin

Carcinogenesis

Catechins

Cell Cycle

Cell Migration

Chili peppers

Colon Cancer

Corn Oil

Cruciferous Vegetables

Cyclooxygenase

Diet

Differentiation

Docosahexaenoic acid

Eicosanoid

Eicosapentaenoic Acid

Ellagic Acid

Epicatechin

Epicatechin gallate

Epidemiology

Epigallocatechin

Epigallocatechin gallate

Epigenetics

Estrogen Receptor

Fatty Acids

Fish

Fish Oil

Flavanols

Food

Gene Polymorphism

Glutathione

Green Tea

Head and Neck Cancer

Hematological Cancer

Hematopoietic stem cells

Heme

Iron

Isothiocyanates

JNK

Leukemia

Liver Cancer

Lung Cancer

Meat

Menopause

Metastasis

Methylxanthines

Mitosis

MnSOD

NADPH

NF-kB

Nutrition

Omega-3

Oxidative stress

Pancreatic Cancer

Phase I Enzyme

Phase II Enzyme

Phenethyl Isothiocyanate

Phytoalexin

Phytochemical

PI-3K/AKT

Polyphenol

PPAR-γ

Progenitor

Progesterone Receptor

Proliferation

Prostate Cancer

Prostate Specific Antigen (PSA)

Reactive Oxygen Species

Red meat

Resveratrol

Retinoic acid

Retinoids

SIRT-1

Skin Cancer

Soy

Stem cells

Sulforaphane

Tea

Theobromine

Theogallin

Theophylline

Thiol

Tumor Initiation

Tumor Progression

Tumor Promotion

Vegetables

Vitamin

Vitamin A

Watercress

Wnt

2

CHAPTER 1

Resveratrol, A Phytoalexin with a Multitude of Anti-Cancer Activities

Richard M. Niles[*] and Gary O. Rankin

Nutrition and Cancer Center, Departments of Biochemistry and Microbiology and Pharmacology, Physiology and Toxicology, Joan C. Edwards School of Medicine, Marshall University, Huntington, WV, USA

Abstract: Resveratrol is a polyphenol produced by certain plants in response to stress. A major dietary source of resveratrol is red wine. This polyphenol has a multitude of effects on mammalian cells, including inhibiting the proliferation and/or inducing apoptosis in cancer cells. This review focuses on recent insights into the metabolism, cancer-specific activities and molecular pathways of resveratrol action. While much work has been published on resveratrol's effects on cancer cells in tissue culture, fewer studies have been performed with rodent cancer models. The animal work shows that resveratrol is effective in inhibiting the development or progression of tumors of the prostate, brain and esophagus. An interesting finding in an animal model of pancreatic cancer is the ability of resveratrol to not only inhibit tumor growth, but to also sensitize the tumor to gemcitabine. Analogous to other phytochemicals, resveratrol inhibits multiple signaling pathways including PI-3K/AKT, NF-kB, TGF-β and COX2 mediated signaling. The major metabolites of resveratrol include piceatannol, resveratrol glucuronide and monosulfated dihydroresveratrol. It is not clear if any of these metabolites have biological activity. There are currently three NCI-registered clinical trials with resveratrol. At present there are no published results from these trials. Low bioavailability of resveratrol may limit its *in vivo* effectiveness. Numerous questions remain to be answered regarding resveratrol's biologic actions and its potential role in the chemoprevention and/or treatment of cancer.

Keywords: Angiogenesis, Apoptosis, Cancer, Cyclooxygenase, Diet, Food, Metastasis, NF-kB, Nutrition, Phase II enzymes, Phytoalexin, PI-3K/AKT, Resveratrol, SIRT-1, Tumor Progression.

INTRODUCTION

Phytoalexins, (alexin from the Greek *alexein*–to ward off or protect) are produced by plants in response to stress such as fungal or microbial infections or environmental stressors such as UV light. These substances fall into three major chemical groups: terpenoids, glycosteroids and alkaloids. One of these phytoalexins, resveratrol (*trans*-3,5,4'-trihydroxystilbene), has received investigative attention for its anti-cancer activity. This is in addition to its well-documented effects on the cardiovascular system [1].

A variety of edible plant components contain resveratrol. However, the highest concentration is found in the skin of grapes. Red wine contains significantly more resveratrol than white wine since the skin of the grapes is left in the fermentation process. Also, the fermentation process appears to either release or concentrate the resveratrol since wine contains considerable more resveratrol than grape juice [2]. The range of resveratrol concentration in wines from around the globe is 1.98–7.13 mg/L [2], although certain varieties and vintage years of Spanish red wines can reach as high as 12.6 mg/L. Another major source of resveratrol is from peanuts. On a per weight basis, peanuts contain, on the average, 50% of the amount of resveratrol found in red wine. Blueberries contain only about 10% of the amount of resveratrol found in an equal weight of grapes. Wines produced from the Pinot Noir variety of grapes contain, on the average, the highest concentration of resveratrol [3].

Resveratrol has a multitude of effects on the biological properties of mammalian cells (Table **1**). These activities range from inducing apoptosis in cancer cells to slowing the progression of diseases such as

*Address Correspondence to Richard M. Niles: Nutrition and Cancer Center and Department of Biochemistry and Microbiology-BBSC 301 Joan C. Edwards School of Medicine, Marshall University, One John Marshall Drive Huntington, WV 25755, USA; E-mail: niles@marshall.edu

Pier Paolo Claudio and Richard M. Niles (Eds)

arthritis and neurological conditions [4]. Recent studies suggest it can mimic the effects of calorie restriction in mice. Specifically, it protected mice against the onset of insulin resistance and early death caused by a high fat/high calorie diet [5] and increased oxidative phosphorylation [6]. Many of these latter effects have been linked to the reported ability of resveratrol to activate sertuin proteins [7]. However, recent experiments have cast concerns over whether resveratrol is a direct activator of SIRT-1 enzyme activity [8]. Apparently, resveratrol reacts with the fluorophore of the SIRT-1 peptide and not directly with unlabeled SIRT-1. This finding suggests that resveratrol mimics the biological effect of calorie restriction through non-sertuin mediated pathways.

In this review, we focus on recent discoveries on the metabolism, cancer-specific activities and molecular pathways of resveratrol. Emphasis is placed on how these findings might be translated into human studies. We end this chapter with some perspectives about resveratrol research and our personal opinions of what is needed to advance this field of research.

Table 1: Biological effects of resveratrol

Cardiovascular	Cancer	Neurological	Aging
Inhibits proliferation of VSMC*	Inhibits proliferation of cancer cells	Reduces brain plaques in animal models of Alzheimer's disease	Increase life span in lower organisms
Stimulates eNOS and vasodilation	Induces phase II enzymes		Activates sertuins??
Inhibits platelet aggregation	Induces apoptosis of cancer cells		Prevents deleterious effects of a high fat diet
Decreases atherogenesis in some animal models	Inhibits invasion and angiogenesis		Increases exercise tolerance
	Inhibits inflammation		

*vascular smooth muscle cells + endothelial nitric oxide synthase.

RESVERATROL AND CANCER

Cell Culture Studies

There have been numerous reports on the ability of resveratrol to affect various properties of different types of cancer cells [9-12] (Table **2**). Most of these earlier studies documented the ability of resveratrol to inhibit cell cycle progression or to induce apoptosis. Recent attention has turned to mechanisms for resveratrol's ability to induce apoptosis and to activate alternate means of inducing cell death. In human colorectal cancer cells, resveratrol activated the caspase-dependent intrinsic pathway through accumulation of mature lysosomal cathepsin D. This study implicates the lysosome as a novel target of resveratrol [13]. Expanding on their initial resveratol work, Trincheri *et al.* reported that resveratrol induces autophagy in DLD1 human colorectal cancer cells [14]. Although this short-term effect of resveratrol was not toxic, chronic (48 h) exposure led to an apoptosis-like cell death.

Chemical analogs of resveratrol (*trans*-resveratrol triacetate, vineatrol, *e*-viniferin and *e*-viniferin pentaacetate) were tested for their biological effects on human colon cancer cells in tissue culture [15]. The rationale for this study was to obtain resveratrol derivatives that have better intestinal absorption and cellular uptake. The *trans*-resveratrol triacetate and vineatrol were as efficient as *trans*-resveratrol in causing the accumulation of the colon cancer cells in the early S phase of the cell cycle. In contrast, *e*-viniferin and its acetylated derivative did not have any measured biological activity on the colon cancer cells. One interesting observation of this study is that resveratrol triacetate and vineatrol significantly enhanced 5-fluorouracil's antiproliferative activity. The next logical step is to determine whether a) the resveratrol triacetate and vineatrol have *in vivo* anti-cancer activity against colon cancer and whether these compounds exhibit increased intestinal absorption in an animal model of colorectal cancer.

In addition to inducing apoptosis and autophagy, resveratrol can also induce a senescence-like state in some human cancer cell lines [16]. The effect was achieved in colon cancer cell lines by using a concentration of resveratrol that do not induce apoptosis. After 10 days of treatment, a large number of cells stained positive for senescence-associated β-galactosidase. This activity of resveratrol is dependent on both p53 and p21 since knockout of these genes dramatically reduced the ability of resveratrol to induce senescence. The authors propose a model in which resveratrol causes an increase in mitochondrial-derived reactive oxygen species and replicative stress resulting in activation of ATM kinase. These two events then lead to activation of p53, followed by an increase in p21 ultimately resulting in senescence.

Resveratrol has been reported to inhibit solid tumor metastasis [17]. Wu *et al.* [18] determined whether HIF-1α might be involved in mediating this activity of resveratrol. They found that resveratrol decreased migration, adhesion, Matrigel invasion activity and MMP-9/2 secretion in Lovo colon carcinoma cells grown under both normoxic and hypoxic conditions. Since resveratrol also reduced the amount of HIF-1α protein under both normoxic and hypoxic conditions, the authors conclude that this decrease likely accounts for the ability of resveratrol to inhibit the *in vitro* invasive activity of these cells. Similar findings were reported by Park *et al.* [19]. This group observed that lysophosphatidic acid (LPA) treatment of human ovarian cancer cells grown under hypoxic conditions resulted in large increases in HIF-1α protein and increased expression of VEGF mRNA and protein. Resveratrol dramatically attenuated the increases in these proteins. Mechanistically, this appeared to be due to an inactivation of the Erk1/2 MAPK pathway and enhanced degradation of HIF-1α protein.

A reversal of doxorubicin resistance in AML cells subsequent to resveratrol treatment was recently reported by Kewon *et al.* [20]. Doxorubicin-resistant AML cell lines were treated with increasing concentrations of resveratrol. This treatment induced growth arrest and apoptotic cell death in a concentration dependent manner. In addition, resveratrol down-regulated the expression of MRP1 (multi-drug resistance protein-1). The expression of this gene was shown to be increased more than 4-fold in the doxorubicin resistant AML cells. These resveratrol-induced changes coincided with a significant increase in the uptake of 5(6)-carboxyfluorescein diacetate, a MRP1 substrate, into the doxorubicin-resistant cells. These data suggest that resveratrol may facilitate the uptake of doxorubicin through down regulation of its efflux pump, MRP1.

Table 2: Resveratrol activity in human cancer cells (2007-2010)

Colon CA	Ovarian CA	AML	Neuroblastoma Xenograft	Pancreatic CA Orthotopic Tumor
Apoptosis/lysosomal cathepsin D	Counteracts hypoxia-induced HIF-1α	Reverses doxorubicin resistance	Reduces growth of xenografted tumors	Enhances the effect of gemcitabine leading to a 75%↓ in tumor volume
autophagy				
senescence				
Inhibition of invasion by ↓ MMP9/2 secretion				

Animal Studies

Although tissue culture studies have provided valuable insights regarding mechanisms through which resveratrol achieves changes in the biology of cancer cells, they can be rather poor predictors of achieving the same biological response from tumors in animals. For example, the authors of this review showed that resveratrol-supplemented mouse chow did not inhibit the growth of a melanoma xenograft in nude mice at any concentration tested. Indeed there was a trend toward increased tumor growth at the higher concentrations of resveratrol [21]. In contrast, the same melanoma cell line in tissue culture responded to resveratrol by undergoing apoptosis at low concentrations of this polyphenol [22]. Fortunately, this latter result appears to be the exception, but relatively few tissue culture reports of resveratrol activity have been followed by animal testing of the same tumor cell line or the ability of resveratrol to inhibit development of the same tumor type in a transgenic model of this disease.

The effect of resveratrol on prostate cancer development has been studied in the TRAMP mouse model. A diet containing 62.5 mg resveratrol per kg AIN-76A diet reduced the incidence of poorly differentiated prostatic adenocarcinoma by 7.7 fold [23]. The effects of resveratrol on regulatory molecules such as IGF-1 were different in the dorsolateral *vs.* the ventral prostate. While poorly differentiated prostate tumors decreased, the number of well-differentiated prostate tumors increased by 42-62% in the resveratrol-fed animals relative to mice receiving the control diet. This indicates that resveratrol is not inhibiting the occurrence of prostate cancer, but rather preventing its progression to a more aggressive form.

Resveratrol was also effective in reducing the growth of human neuroblastoma xenografts in nude mice. A reduction of up to 80% was achieved when the mice were given up to 50 mg/kg of resveratrol by gavage daily for five weeks. The serum resveratrol concentration was 2-10 µmol/L, but no detectable amounts of this polypheno were found in the xenografted tumor. In addition, peri-tumoral injections of 5 mg of resveratrol over 16 days resulted in rapid tumor regression [24]. Since resveratrol was not detectable in the tumors, there remains the possibility that one of the resveratrol metabolites, such as piceatannol, or resveratrol glucuronide, might be the component responsible for the inhibition of tumor growth.

A more pharmaceutical drug approach was taken by Narayanan *et al.* [25]. This group used PTEN knock out mice as a model of prostate cancer. Resveratrol was encapsulated in liposomes and either given individually or in combination with liposome-encapsulated curcumin by oral gavage. The combinations of liposome encapsulated curcumin and resveratrol significantly inhibited the incidence of prostatic adenocarcinomas by 75% and decreased prostate weight by ~50%. The combination of liposomal curcumin and resveratrol greatly enhances the plasma levels of both compounds. The results of these experiments suggest that combining several dietary constituents and also lipid encapsulation enhances absorption and the anti-tumor activity of both compounds.

An interesting model to study the cancer chemoprevention ability of resveratrol is Barrett's esophageal metaplasia, a pre-neoplastic condition that progresses at a certain rate to invasive adenocarcinoma. Woodall *et al.* [26] used a rat model of esophagoduodenal anastomosis. Rats were treated with 7 mg/kg resveratrol *via* intraperitoneal injection. Thirty-one rats in the 5-month resveratrol group had decreased severity of esophagitis. There was also a decreased incidence of intestinal metaplasia and incidence of carcinoma as compared to the saline treated groups. This proof of concept paves the way for more detailed investigation of resveratrol's chemoprevention effects at low dietary levels of resveratrol.

Pancreatic cancer has a dismal five year survival rate due in part to the failure of early detection of this malignancy. Presently, gemcitabine is the standard of care for patients with advanced disease. However, this drug has not significantly prolonged survival in this population of patients. Harikumar *et al.* [27] tested the ability of resveratrol to enhance the activity of gemcitabine. They used an orthotopic model of human pancreatic cancer where the human pancreatic cell line MIA PaCa-2 was implanted into the subcapsular region of the pancreas. After a week of recovery, mice were randomized to groups where they received resveratrol at 40 mg/kg p.o. daily, gemcitabine alone at 25 mg/kg i.p. twice per week, or a combination of the resveratrol and gemcitabine treatments. Surprisingly resveratrol inhibited tumor growth (50% of control group) to the same extent as gemcitabine. The combination of the two agents resulted in a further decrease in tumor volume to a 75% reduction relative to the control group. The authors speculate that the ability of resveratrol to inhibit NF-kB activity is important for its biological activity in pancreatic cancer. However, since resveratrol acts in a pleiotropic fashion, other targets or a combination of multiple targets may contribute to its anti-cancer activity. There is a growing body of literature that a number of dietary agents can potentiate the activity of cancer chemotherapeutic agents. However this is the first report that resveratrol is an effective anti-tumor agent in an orthotopic model of human pancreatic cancer and raises the possibility that dietary agents may play a role in either the prevention, or treatment in combination with chemotherapy, of this intractable malignancy.

Molecular Pathways

In light of the cancer inhibitory/apoptosis inducing effects of resveratrol, there has been a high amount of interest in the molecular pathways that mediate these biological changes. Fig. **1** illustrates the activity of resveratrol on multiple signaling pathways. In human multiple myeloma cells, resveratrol inhibits proliferation, induces apoptosis, and overcomes resistance to certain chemotherapy agents [28]. As might be predicted, various proliferative and anti-apoptotic gene products were down-regulated such as cyclin D1, XIAP, survivin, Bcl-2, *etc.* However, looking upstream of these changes in protein expression, the authors found that resveratrol suppressed the constitutively active NF-kB through inhibition of IkBα kinase and the phosphorylation of IkBα and p65. This phytoalexin also inhibited both constitutive and IL-6 induced activation of STAT3. Lastly, it was shown that resveratrol suppressed constitutively active AKT. Exactly how resveratrol was able to accomplish these changes in AKT and IKK was not addressed in this study.

The PI-3Kinase and AKT pathways were also implicated in the growth inhibitory and apoptosis-inducing effects of resveratrol in human prostate tumor cells [29]. This action of resveratrol was androgen receptor and estrogen receptor-α dependent and correlated with GSK-3 dephosphorylation and decreased cyclin D1 levels. Importantly, this effect was also noted in primary cells cultured from human prostate tumors. The authors speculate that resveratrol inhibits the non-genomic interaction between the steroid hormone receptors and PI-3 kinase. Following on the PI-3kinase theme, Frojdo *et al.* [30] found that resveratrol is a class IA phosphoinositide 3-kinase inhibitor. This work was performed in both "test-tube" assays and in cultured muscle cell lines. Resveratrol interacted with the ATP binding site of class IA PI-3kinase in a competitive and reversible manner. The class IA PI-3 kinases are of the p85/100 variety and mediate mitogenic signaling and survival pathways. The class IB PI-3 kinases are activated by G-protein coupled receptors and are involved in immune responses. However, it remains to be determined whether resveratrol inhibits PI-3 kinase in the context of the cellular environment found in a variety of human cancer cells.

A broader approach to unraveling the molecular mechanism of the anti-proliferative action of resveratrol in lung cancer cells was taken by Whyte *et al.* [31]. They used microarray gene expression profiling and high through-put immunoblotting (Power Blots) to identify genes and proteins whose expression is altered in resveratrol-treated A549 lung cancer cells. The authors identified 127 protein bands that had a fold change of 1.25 or higher in resveratrol-treated *vs.* control cells. Analysis of 47,500 transcripts identified 5,916 genes whose expression was altered by 1.2 fold in the resveratrol-treated cells compared to control cells. Ingenuity Pathway Analysis identified G1-S cell cycle check point and G2-M cell cycle checkpoint pathways as well as cell apoptosis pathways to be activated by resveratrol. Also TGF–β components were found altered by resveratrol treatment. Specifically, Smad2 and 4 were found to be down-regulated while Smad 7 was found to be up-regulated in resveratrol-treated cells. Lastly, the NF-kB and p38 MAPK pathways were shown to be altered by resveratrol. However, statistical methods applied to these assays were limited and it is not clear how many of the protein and gene expression changes are truly significant given the relatively small number of repeat experiments (not replicates in the same experiments). Nonetheless, the changes in these pathways are logical given the documented biological activity of resveratrol.

A different target for resveratrol was identified by Zykova *et al.* [32]. These authors found that resveratrol directly binds to COX-2 and that this binding is required for resveratrol to inhibit anchorage-independent growth of the human colon adenocarcinoma HT-29 cell line. This binding correlated with the ability of resveratrol to inhibit COX-2-mediated PGE2 production. An important finding was that cells deficient in COX-2 did not respond to resveratrol by decreasing their proliferation. However, it was not determined if the COX-2 deficient cells also were resistant to the ability of resveratrol to inhibit anchorage-independent growth (colony formation in soft agarose).

Although resveratrol can induce autophagy in cancer cells, treatment of non-malignant cells such as NIH 3T3 and HEK 293 cells with resveratrol attenuated autophagy that was induced in response to nutrient deprivation or the mTOR inhibitor rapamycin. This action of resveratrol was shown to be independent of SIRT1 [33]. A large scale kinase screen identified p70 S6 kinase as a target of resveratrol. Blocking the activity of S6 kinase by other means such as a dominant-negative mutant or RNAi also resulted in disruption of autophagy. The mechanism of resveratrol's ability to inhibit S6 kinase was not explored in this study. The authors note that both resveratrol treated and S6K1-/-mice have less body fat and their peripheral tissues remain highly sensitive to insulin. Also, mitochondrial number and activity are increased in both S6K1-/-and resveratrol-treated mice. These observations suggest that resveratrol's ability to inhibit S6 kinase might account for some of its physiological effects.

Further evidence for the effect of resveratrol on NF-kB activity was recently obtained by Benitez *et al.* [34]. In PC-3 human prostate cancer cells, resveratrol induced a dose-dependent cytoplasmic retention of NF-kB, which resulted in the inhibition of NF-kB-mediated transcriptional activity induced by EGF and TNFα. A similar strong effect of resveratrol was not seen in LNCaP cells. It appears that this cytoplasmic retention of NF-kB is caused by a resveratrol-induced increase in the level of IkBα. The differences in response to resveratrol between PC-3 and LNCaP may be due to PC-3's being AR⁻and ERα⁺, while LNCaP cells are AR⁺ and ERα⁻. One concern about this study is that the authors showed that at low concentrations (10 μM or less), resveratrol stimulated NF-kB activity, while at high concentrations it inhibited the activity of this transcription factor. Since the level of resveratrol likely to reach tumors *in vivo* will be well below 10 μM, it raises the possibility that stimulation of NF-kB activity could occur in certain prostate cancers. If this occurred, it might enhance survival of the cancer cells and render them more resistant to chemotherapeutic drugs.

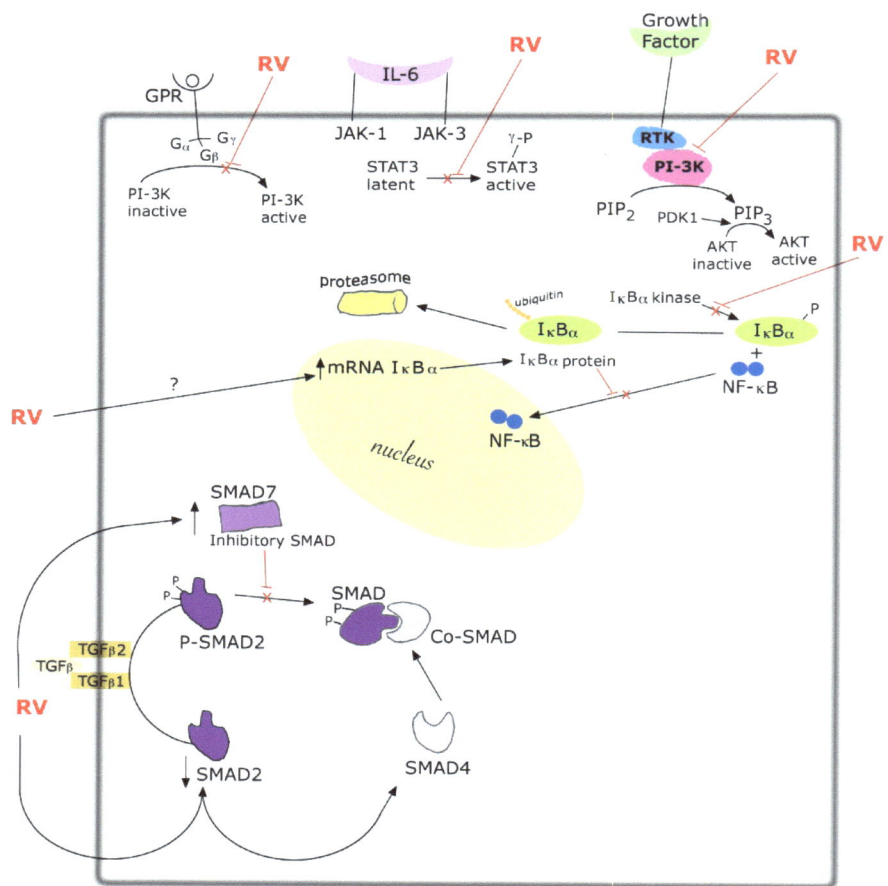

Figure 1: Resveratrol affects the activity of multiple signaling pathways.

This diagram illustrates the inhibitory effect of resveratrol (RV) on multiple signaling pathways. These include G-protein coupled receptor mediated stimulation of PI-3K activity; interleukin-mediated conversion of latent to active STAT3; inhibition of PI-3K activity to prevent activation of AKT; inhibition of IκBα kinase activity to prevent migration of NF-κB into the nucleus; stimulation of the inhibitory SMAD7 to prevent phosphorylated SMAD2 from binding with the co-SMAD4 thus disrupting TGFβ stimulation of target genes. RV also stimulates an increase in the mRNA encoding IκBα preventing "free" NF-κB from entering the nucleus. The mechanism/pathway by which RV stimulates the expression of the IκBα gene is not known.

PHARMACOKINETICS AND BIOTRANSFORMATION

Pharmacokinetics

The pharmacokinetics of trans-resveratrol (Fig. **2**) has been studied in detail in animals [21, 35, 36] and humans [37–40]. In these studies, it was found that resveratrol was well absorbed from the gastrointestinal tract, but bioavailability was extremely low, primarily due to rapid and extensive biotransformation in the liver, gastrointestinal epithelial cells, and possibly other tissues [41]. Excretion of resveratrol and its metabolites is primarily *via* the urine and feces, with the majority (up to 85%) of the administered dose appearing in urine as metabolites [38].

In animal studies, peak plasma resveratrol levels are obtained in rats between five and ten minutes following oral administration with a plasma elimination $T_{1/2}$ between 12 and 15 minutes [35]. Resveratrol is well absorbed following oral administration in rats with 50-75% of the dose absorbed from the gastrointestinal tract [42]. In athymic (Nu/Nu) mice, an oral bolus of 75 mg/kg resveratrol resulted in plasma, skin and liver levels respectively of resveratrol: 28.4, 21.2 and 73.0 μM; resveratrol glucuronide: 36.4, 4.7 and 78.8 μM and piceatannol: 5.3, 2.4 and 11.5 μM at five minutes post-treatment. Resveratrol was also distributed to melanoma tumors at five minutes post-oral administration in tumor-bearing athymic mice, but tumor resveratrol levels were only about 10% of plasma levels and less than half the level of surrounding skin [21]. Similar low plasma levels and rapid clearance of resveratrol have been observed in other animal studies [43–46].

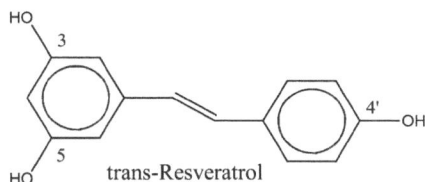

Figure 2: Chemical structure of *trans*-resveratrol.

In humans, resveratrol also exhibits high absorption, but very low bioavailability when administered orally. Vitaglione *et al.* [39] examined resveratrol bioavailability from red wine in 25 healthy volunteers, but found only trace amounts of resveratrol in plasma 30 minutes after consumption. Walle *et al.* [38] examined the pharmacokinetics of ^{14}C-resveratrol in six healthy human volunteers. When a 25 mg oral dose was administered, absorption was ≥ 70%; the total peak resveratrol level (resveratrol plus metabolites) was 491 ng/ml, and the plasma $T_{1/2}$ was about 9 hr. However, the plasma level of the unmetabolized resveratrol was only < 5 ng/ml, supporting a low bioavailability for the parent resveratrol. Boocock *et al.* [40] determined the pharmacokinetics of orally administered resveratrol (0.5–5 g) and three metabolites in ten volunteers. They also determined that resveratrol had a plasma $T_{1/2}$ of ~ 9 hr, and at the highest dose, peak plasma levels (539 ng/ml) occurred between 0.83 and 1.5 hr post-administration. In addition, a second plasma peak of resveratrol was observed around 5 hr post-dosing, which was interpreted as evidence of enterohepatic cycling for resveratrol, a finding also observed in rats [42]. Vaz-da-Silva *et al.* [47] studied the effect of food intake on resveratrol pharmacokinetics in 24 healthy human volunteers. They noted that food reduced the bioavailability of resveratrol and delayed the time to peak concentration from 0.5 hr in fasted subjects to 2.0 hr in fed subjects. Thus, as observed in animal studies, humans have high absorption of resveratrol but rapid clearance from the plasma.

Metabolism

The rapid clearance (low bioavailability) of resveratrol is due primarily to extensive hepatic and gastrointestinal metabolism. To date, four biotransformation pathways have been identified in animals and/or humans (Fig. **3**). The relative contributions of each pathway vary somewhat depending on species, dose and model used, but the major metabolites of resveratrol resulting from Phase II metabolism are: sulfation and glucuronidation.

The two Phase I metabolites of trans-resveratrol that have been identified are dihydroresveratrol (reduction) and piceatannol (oxidation) (Fig. **3**). Walle *et al.* [38] qualitatively detected both a monoglucuronide and a monosulfate conjugate of dihydroresveratrol in the urine of humans treated orally with 100 mg resveratrol. The origins of the reduction of the double bond were not determined with certainty, but it was hypothesized that intestinal microflora might be responsible from this reduction. Dihydroresveratrol and its monsulfate conjugate have also been identified in the urine of resveratrol-treated rats [48]. Piceatannol results from the cytochrome P450 (CYP)-mediated oxidation of trans-resveratrol at the 3' position. This oxidation can occur naturally in plants (*e.g.* grapes) and is seen in some animal and human studies [21, 49, 50] but not others [43]. In humans, the primary CYPs responsible for oxidation of trans-resveratrol to picatannol are CYP1B1 and CYP1A2 [49, 50].

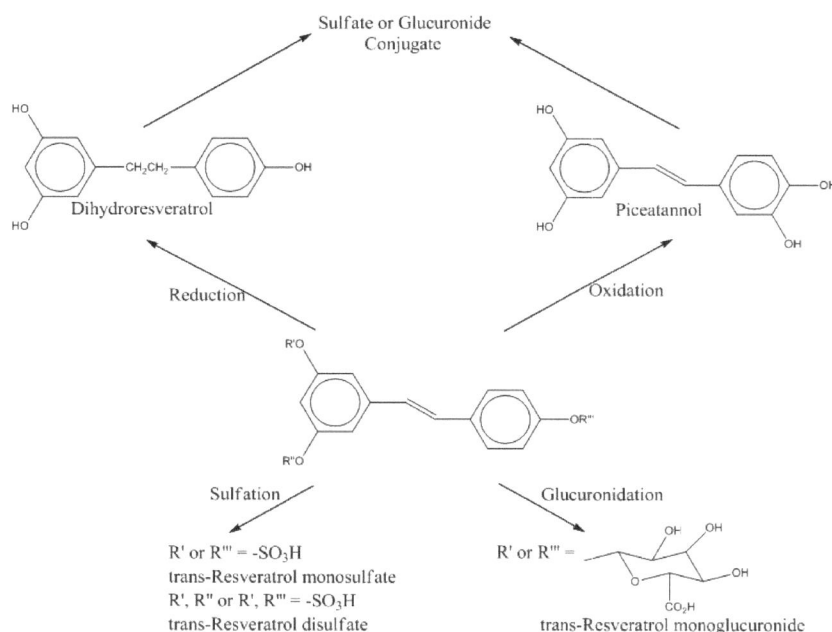

Figure 3: Biotransformation of *trans*-resveratrol.

The major trans-resveratrol metabolites in animals and humans are Phase II metabolites resulting from sulfation or glucuronidation of one or more of the phenolic hydroxyl groups in liver and/or intestine. These metabolites are formed *in vitro* (43) and *in vivo* [36, 38, 40, 51]. Several sulfate and/or glucuronide conjugates of trans-resveratrol have been identified in human plasma or urine including the 3-sulfate, 3, 4'-disulfate, 3, 5-disulfate, 3-glucuronide, and 4'-glucuronide, with the sulfates being the predominant conjugates [40, 51]. trans-Resveratrol diglucuronides have also been detected in human plasma and urine as minor metabolites [51]. Sulfation of trans-resveratrol is catalyzed primarily by the human cytosolic sulfotransferase SULT1A1 and SULT1E1 isozymes [38, 52]. Glucuronidation of trans-resveratrol also occurs in human intestine and liver and is catalyzed by the UDP—glucuronosyl transferases UGT1A1 and

UGT1A9, with minor contributions from UGT1A10 [53]. The major site of monosulfate and monoglucuronide conjugation occurs at the 3-position of trans-resveratrol [51, 53]. The glucuronide conjugates and, to a lesser extent, the sulfate conjugates are also substrates for the canalicular transporter Mrp2, which would facilitate conjugate elimination into bile [54].

CLINICAL TRIALS

A search of the National Cancer Institute's data base on registered clinical trials yielded three currently active human trials that involve resveratrol, or one of its chemical derivatives. One trial (NCT00256334) being conducted by the Chao Family Comprehensive Cancer Center at the University of California at Irvine, with Randall Holcombe, MD as P.I., involves administering resveratrol to patients with confirmed colon cancer. The study is classified as a Phase I/II trial and is based on the PI's laboratory work showing that resveratrol modulates the Wnt signaling pathway that is highly active in 85% of sporadic colon cancer. The study will look at biomarkers, presumably Wnt activity, in specimens from the patient's tumor and normal mucosa.

A second trial (NCT00455416) is studying a dietary intervention in patients with Follicular Lymphoma. The P.I. is Harald Holte, MD, Ph.D. at the Rikshospitalet University Hospital in Norway. It appears that resveratrol may only be one of several dietary constituents to be tested in this study. It is classified as a Phase II clinical study that seeks to enroll 45 patients. The aim is to determine whether the dietary intervention affects the rate of apoptosis, proliferation and immune cell infiltrates in the patient's cancer.

The third NCI-registered trial (NCT00920556) aims to assess the safety and activity of SRT501, an analog of resveratrol with improved bioavailability relative to the parent molecule. This compound will be tested alone or in combination with Borezomib (a proteosomal inhibitor) in patients with multiple myeloma. This is a phase II trial conducted by GlaxoSmithKline. This study will determine the safety and tolerability of SRT501 (5.0g) and define objective responses and time to progression of the multiple myeloma. A sub-group of 15 patients will participate in a side study to assess the pharmacokinetics of SRT501.

All of these trials are ongoing and still enrolling patients. At the time of the writing of this chapter there were no published results from these trials. In light of the increasing number of animal studies documenting the effectiveness of resveratrol in preventing or inhibiting the growth of established specific tumors, it is likely that additional clinical trials will be initiated over the next several years.

PERSPECTIVES AND OPINIONS

Studies conducted over the last three years, together with those published previously, clearly show that resveratrol has multiple targets resulting in a variety of cellular changes. Despite this diversity, there are a few common themes. In a number of different tumor types, resveratrol decreases the activity of the PI-3K, AKT, NF-kB pathway. The mechanism by which resveratrol inhibits this pathway might be different in various cancer cells, but the effect is to arrest growth and induce apoptosis. There continues to be a strong need to follow-up the effects of resveratrol on cancer cell growth, apoptosis, *etc.* in cell culture with animal studies. Choosing the appropriate animal model is critical. Testing of chemoprevention will require transgenic animal models that recapitulate most aspects of the development of the same type of cancer in humans. Measuring the effect of resveratrol on established tumor growth, invasion/metastasis might be best accomplished with orthotopic injections of tumor cells. These animal studies should include pharmacokinetics of resveratrol metabolism, elimination, and concentration in plasma and tumor.

Future studies might consider using resveratrol in combination with other dietary constituents, such as other phytochemicals found in red wine (quercetin, for example). Also, since pure resveratrol is rapidly oxidized, it would be interesting to combine this phytoalexin with anti-oxidants such as vitamin C or vitamin E. Lastly, pharmacokinetic studies suggest that resveratrol is rapidly metabolized to piceatannol, resveratrol glucuronide and resveratrol sulfate. We need to know whether any of these metabolites have biological activity, since published studies generally agree that the concentration of the parent compound in plasma and tumor tissue is much lower than what is used in tissue culture studies. Since studies have shown significant effects of resveratrol in slowing progression of prostate and colon cancer in animal models, one must conclude that either low concentrations of resveratrol are more effective *in vivo* (*i.e.* small doses over a prolonged period of time), or that a resveratrol metabolite is the active biological molecule.

The authors suggest that current and future researchers in this field consider our suggestions and ponder our questions …… over a glass of red wine!

REFERENCES

[1]   Bertelli AA, Das KK. Grapes, wine, resveratrol and heart health. J Cardiovasc Pharmacol 2009; 54: 468-76.

[2]   Roy H, Lundy S. Pennington Nutrition Series #7 2005.

[3]   Stervbo U, Vang O, Bonneser CA. Review of the content of the putative chemopreventive phytoalexin resveratrol in red wine. Food Chemistry 2007; 101: 449-59.

[4]   Harlkumar KB, Aggarwal BB. Resveratrol, a multi-targeted agent for age-associated chronic disease. Cell Cycle 2008; 7: 1020-37.

[5]   Bauer JA, Pearson KJ, Price NL, Jamieson HA, *et al.* Resveratrol improves health and survival of mice on high calorie diet. Nature 444 2006; 444: 337-42.

[6]   Lagouge M, Argmann C, Gerhardt-Hines Z, Meziane H, *et al.* Resveratrol improves mitochondrial function and protects against metabolic disease by activating SIRT1 and PGC-1α. Cell 2006; 127: 1109-22.

[7]   Howitz KT, Litterman KJ, Cohen HY, Lamming DW, *et al.* Small molecule activators of sirtuins extend *Saccharomyces cerevisiae* lifespan. Nature 2003; 425: 191-96.

[8]   Beher D, Wy J, Cumine S, Kim KW, *et al.* Regulation of cell survival by resveratrol involves inhibition of NF-kB-regulated gene expression in prostate cancer cells. The Prostate 2009; 69: 1045-54.

[9]   Schneider Y, Vincent F, Duranton B, Badolo L, *et al.* Anti-proliferative effect of resveratrol, a natural component of grapes and wine, on human colonic cancer cells. Cancer Lett 2000; 158: 85-91.

[10]   Dorrie J, Gerauer H, Wachter Y, Zunino SJ. Resveratrol induces extensive apoptosis by depolarizing mitochondrial membranes and activating caspase-9 in acute lymphoblastic leukemia cells. Cancer Res 2001; 61: 4731-39.

[11]   Damianaki A, Bakogeorgou E, Kampa M, Notas G, *et al.* Potent inhibitory action of red wine polyphenols on human breast cancer cells. J Cell Biochem 2000; 78: 429-41.

[12]   Hsieh TC, Wu JM. Differential effects on growth, cell cycle arrest, and induction of apoptosis by resveratrol in human prostate cancer cell lines. Exp Cell Res 1999; 249: 109-15.

[13]   Trincheri NF, Nicotra G, Follo C, Castio R. Isidoro C. Resveratrol induces cell death in colorectal cancer cells by a novel pathway involving lysosomal cathepsin D. Carcinogenesis 2007; 28: 922-31.

[14]   Trincheri NF, Follo C, Nocotra G, Peracchio C, *et al.* Resveratrol-induced apoptosis depends on the lipid kinase activity of Vps34 and on the formation of autophagolysosomes. Carcinogenesis 2008; 29: 381-89.

[15]   Colin D, Gimazane A, Lizard G, Isard J-C, *et al.* Effects of resveratrol analogs on cell cycle progression, cell cycle associated proteins and 5-fluorouracil sensitivity in human derived colon cancer cells. Int J Cancer 2009; 124: 2780-88.

[16]   Heiss EH, Schilder YDC, Dirsch VM. Chronic treatment with resveratrol induces redox stress-and Ataxia Telangiectasia-mutated (ATM)-dependent senescence in p53-positive cancer cells. J Biol Chem 2007; 282: 26759-66.

[17]   Busquets S, Ametler E, Fuster G, *et al.* Resveratrol, a natural diphenol, reduces metastatic growth in an experimental cancer model. Cancer Lett 2007; 245: 144-48.

[18]   Wu H, Liang X, Fang Y, Qin X, Zhang Y, Liu J. Resveratrol inhibits hypoxia-induced metastasis potential enhancement by restricting hypoxia-induced factor-1a expression in colon carcinoma cells. Biomed Pharmacother 2008; 62: 613-21.

[19]   Park SY, Jeong KJ, Yoon DS, Choi WS, *et al.* Hypoxia enhances LPA_induced HIF-1α and VEGF expression: their inhibition by resveratrol. Cancer Lett 2007; 258: 63-9.

[20]   Kweon SH, Song JH, Kim TS. Resveratrol-mediated reversal of doxorubicin resistance in acute myeloid leukemia cells *via* downregulation of MRP1 expression. Biochem Biophys Res Comm Epub, March 2010.

[21]   Niles RM, Cook CP, Meadows G.G, Fu UM, McLaughlin JL, Rankin GO. Resveratrol is rapidly metabolized in athymimc (nu/nu) mice and does not inhibit human melanoma xenograft tumor growth. J. Nutrition 2006;135: 2542-46.

[22]   Niles RM, McFarland M, Weimer MB, Redkar A, Fu Y-M, Meadows GG. Resveratrol is a potent inducer of apoptosis in human melanoma cells. Cancer Lett 2003; 190: 1157-63.

[23]   Harper CF, Patel BB, Wang J, *et al.* Resveratrol suppresses prostate cancer progression in transgenic mice. Carcinogenesis 2007; 28: 1946-53.

[24]   Van Gingel PR, Sareen D, Subramanian L, *et al.* Resveratrol inhibits tumor growth of human neuroblastoma and mediates apoptosis by directly targeting mitochondria. Clin Cancer Res 2007; 13: 5162-69.

[25]   Naranyanan NK, Nargi D, Randolph C, Naraaynan BA. Liposome encapsulation of curcumin and resveratrol in combination reduces prostate cancer incidence in PTEN knockout mice. Int J Cancer 2009; 125: 1-8.

[26]   Woodall CE, Li Y, Liu QH, Wo J, Martin RCG. Chemoprevention of metaplasia initiation and carcinogenic progression to esophageal adenocarcinoma by resveratrol supplementation. Anti-Cancer Drugs 2009; 20: 437-43.

[27]   Harikumar KB, Kunnumakkara AB, Sethi G, *et al.* Resveratrol, a multi-targeted agent, can enhance antitumor activity of gemcitabine *in vitro* and in an orthotopic mouse model of human pancreatic cancer. Int J Cancer 2009; 127: 257-268.

[28]   Bhardwaj A, Sethi G, Vadhan-Raj S, *et al.* Resveratrol inhibits proliferation, induces apoptosis, and overcomes chemoresistance through down-regulation of STAT3 and nuclear factor-kB-regulated antiapoptotic and cell survival gene products in human multiple myeloma cells. Blood 2007; 109: 2293-2302.

[29]   Benitez DA, Pozo-Guisado E, Clementi, M, Castellon E, Fernandez-Salguero PM. Non-genomic action of resveratrol on androgen and oestrogen receptors in prostate cancer: modulation of the phosphoinositide 3-kinase pathway. Brit J Cancer 2007 96: 595-604.

[30]   Frojdo S, Cozzone D, Vidal H, Pirola L. Resveratrol is a class IA phosphoinositide 3-kinase inhibitor. Biochem J 2007; 406: 511-18.

[31]   Whyte L, Huang Y-Y, Torres K, Metha RG. Molecular mechanisms of resveratrol action in lung cancer cells using dual protein and microarray analyses. Cancer Res 2007; 67: 12007-17.

[32]   Zykova TA, Zhu F, Zhai X, *et al.* Resveratrol directly targets COX-2 to inhibit carcinogenesis. Mol Carcinogenesis 2008; 47: 797-805.

[33]   Armour SM, Baur JA, Hsieh SM, *et al.* Inhibition of mammalian S6 kinase by resveratrol suppresses autophagy. Aging 2009; 1:515-28.

[34]   Benitez DA, Hermoso MA, Pozo-Guidado E, Fernandez-Salguero PM, Castellon EA. Regulation of cell survival by resveratrol involves inhibition of NF-kappa B-regulated gene expression in prostate cancer cells. Prostate 2009; 69: 1045-54.

[35]   Gescher AJ, Steward WP. Relationship between mechanisms, bioavailability, and preclinical chemoprevention efficacy of resveratrol: A conundrum. Cancer Epidemiol Biomarkers Prev 2003; 12: 953-57.

[36]   Abd El-Mohsen M, Bayele H, Kuhnle G, *et al.* Distribution of [³H]trans-resveratrol in rat tissues following oral administration. Br J Nutr 2006; 96: 62-70.

[37]   Goldberg DM, Yan J, Soleas GJ. Absorption of three wine-related polyphenols in three different matrices by healthy subjects. Clin Biochem 2003; 36: 79-87.

[38]   Walle T, Hsieh F, DeLegge MH, Oatis JE, Jr, Walle UK. High absorption but very low bioavailability of oral resveratrol in humans. Drug Metab Dispos 2004; 32: 1377-82.

[39]   Vitaglione P, Sforza S, Galaverna G, Ghidini C, Caporaso N, Vescovi PP, Fogliano V, Marchelli R. Bioavailability of trans-resveratrol from red wine in humans. Mol Nutr Food Res 2005; 49: 495-504.

[40]   Boocock DJ, Faust GES, Patel KR, *et al.* Phase I dose escalation pharmacokinetic study in healthy volunteers of resveratrol, a potential cancer chemopreventive agent. Cancer Epidemiol Biomarkers Prev 2007; 16: 1246-52.

[41]   Wenzel E, Somoza V. Metabolism and bioavailability of trans-resveratrol. Mol Nutr Food Res 2005; 49: 472-81.

[42]   Soleas GJ, Angelini M, Grass L, Diamandis EP, Goldberg DM. Absorption of trans-resveratrol in rats. Methods Enzymol 2001; 335: 145-54.

[43]   Yu C, Shin YG, Chow A, Li Y, *et al.* Human, rat, and mouse metabolism of resveratrol. Pharm Res 2002; 19: 1907-14.

[44]   Juan ME, Vindardell, MP, Planas JM. The daily oral administration of high doses of trans-resveratrol to rats for 28 days is not harmful. J Nutr. 2002: 132 257-60.

[45]   Asensi M, Medina I, Ortega A, *et al.* Inhibition of cancer growth by resveratrol is related to its low bioavailability. Free Radic Biol Med 2002; 33: 387-98.

[46]   Sale S, Verschoyle RD, Boocock D, *et al.* Pharmacokinetics in mice and growth-inhibitory properties of the putative cancer chemopreventative agent resveratrol and the synthetic analogue 3,4,5,4'-tetramethoxystilbene. Br J Cancer 2004; 9: 736-44.

[47] Vaz-da-Silva M, Loureiro AL, Falcao A, *et al.* Effect of food on the pharmacokinetic profile of trans-resveratrol. Int J Clin Pharmacol Ther 2008; 46: 564-70.

[48] Wang D, Hang T, Wu C, Lui W. Identification of the major metabolites of resveratrol in rat urine by HPLC-MS/MS. J Chromatogr B Analyt Technol Biomed Life Sci 2005; 829: 97-106.

[49] Potter GA, Patterson LH, Wanogho EP, *et al.* The cancer preventative agent resveratrol is converted to the anticancer agent piceatannol by the cytochrome P450 enzyme CYP1B1. Br J Cancer 2002; 86: 774-77.

[50] Piver B, Fer M, Vitrac X, Merrillon JM, Dreano Y, Berthou F, Lucas D. Involvement of cytochrome P450 1A2 in the biotransformation of trans-resveratrol in human liver microsomes. Biochem Pharmacol 2004; 68: 773-82.

[51] Burkon A, Somoza V. Quantification of free and protein-bound trans-resveratrol metabolites and identification of trans-resveratrol-C/O-conjugated diglucuronides–two novel resveratrol metabolites in human plasma. Mol Nutr Food Res 2008; 52: 549-57.

[52] Ung D, Nagar S. Variable sulfation of dietary polyphenols by recombinant human sulfotransferase (SULT) 1A1 genetic variants and SULT1E1. Drug Metab Dispos. 2007; 35: 740-46.

[53] Iwuchukwu OF, Nagar S. Resveratrol (trans-resveratrol, 3,5,4'-trihydroxy-trans-stilbene) glucuronidation exhibits atypical enzyme kinetics in various protein sources. Drug Metab Dispos. 2008; 36: 322-30.

[54] Maier-Salamon A, Hagenauer B, Reznicek G, Szekeres T, Thalhammer T, Jager W. Metabolism and disposition of resveratrol in the isolated perfused rat liver: role of Mrp2 in the biliary excretion of glucuronides. J Pharm Sci. 2008; 97: 1615-28.

Nutrition and Cancer, From Epidemiology to Biology, 2013, 15-25

CHAPTER 2

Capsaicin: Potential Applications in Cancer Therapy

Jamie K. Lau[$], Kathleen C. Brown[$], Aaron M. Dom and Piyali Dasgupta[*]

Nutrition and Cancer Center, Department of Pharmacology, Physiology, and Toxicology, Joan C. Edwards School of Medicine, Marshall University, Huntington, WV, USA

Abstract: Capsaicin is an active ingredient of chili peppers. Although traditionally associated with chemopreventive and anti-carcinogenic activity, recent studies have shown that capsaicin has profound anti-neoplastic effects in several types of human cancer cells. The biological activity of capsaicin is mediated by the transient receptor potential vanilloid [TRPV] superfamily of ion channel receptors. Specifically, capsaicin is an agonist of the TRPV1 receptor. The growth-inhibitory properties of capsaicin have been found to be mediated by TRPV1-dependent and independent mechanisms. Experiments in multiple animal models have demonstrated that the anti-cancer activity of capsaicin is not associated with any discomfort or toxicity. The present review summarizes the current knowledge on the growth-inhibitory activity of capsaicin and discusses the signaling pathways underlying its anti-cancer effects. Future studies involving the design of capsaicin-mimetics with improved selectivity may represent novel strategies in the treatment of human cancers.

Keywords: Angiogenesis, Apoptosis, Autophagy, Breast Cancer, Cancer, Capsaicin, Cell Cycle, Cell Migration, Chili Peppers, Colon Cancer, Diet, Food, Lung Cancer, Nutrition, Prostate Cancer.

INTRODUCTION

Capsaicin (trans-8-methyl-N-vanillyl-6-noneamide) is the principal, pungent ingredient of chili peppers of the plant genus *Capsicum solanaceae* (Fig. **1**). It is used topically to treat pain and inflammation associated with a variety of diseases [1]. However, emerging evidence shows that it can induce apoptosis in multiple transformed cell types *in vitro* and in animal models of carcinogenesis [2]. Capsaicin has also been shown to induce apoptosis in non-small cell lung cancer cells (NSCLCs), T-cell leukemia cells, esophageal carcinoma cells, astroglioma cells, and prostate, colon and gastric cancer cells in cell culture models [3-9]. In nude mice models of prostate cancer, the administration of capsaicin has been shown to suppress tumor growth [8-15].

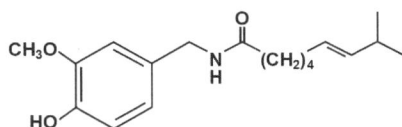

Figure 1: The molecular structure of capsaicin (trans-8-methyl-N-vanillyl-6-noneamide).

Capsaicin has been known to be responsible for the so-called "heat sensation" or "burning sensation" experienced upon ingestion of chili peppers [16]. This "heat-sensation" is responsible for the spiciness of capsaicin and arises due to the binding of capsaicin to transient receptor potential vanilloid (TRPV) ion-channel receptors [17, 18]. This binding activity produces depolarization of sensory neurons [18]. Therefore, capsaicin does not cause any "chemical burn" or "tissue damage;" it only causes the sensation of one.

The ability of capsaicin to produce a "heat-sensation" in humans has often raised concerns about its use as an anti-cancer drug [19]. The "degree of hotness," or the comparative capsaicin level, is conventionally

*Address Correspondence to Piyali Dasgupta: Nutrition and Cancer Center, Department of Pharmacology, Physiology and Toxicology, Joan C. Edwards School of Medicine, Marshall University, Byrd Biotechnology Science Center, Room 335G, 1700 Third Avenue, Huntington WV, 25755, USA; E-mail: dasgupta@marshall.edu
[$]These two authors contributed equally to this work.

Pier Paolo Claudio and Richard M. Niles (Eds)

measured on the Scoville Scale (http://www.chilliworld.com/FactFile/Scoville_Scale.asp). Each Scoville Unit measures 1/15 parts per million of capsaicin in a chili pepper (Fig. **2**).

A survey of existing literature shows that researchers have used wide ranging doses of capsaicin in different animal model systems and have reported no signs of irritation to animals. Similarly, capsaicin has been administered to animals *via* many methods and no discomfort was observed. Table **1** lists the concentration of capsaicin used by laboratories for anti-cancer research or chemoprevention studies. Erin *et al.* (2006) administered an extremely high dose of 150 mg/kg capsaicin to mice to inactivate neurons [20]. Their mice did not show any signs of gross toxicity. Therefore, it may be envisaged that capsaicin could be a safe nutritional agent for cancer therapy and management in humans. Cancer statistics show that the incidence of lung cancer, breast cancer and prostate cancer is lower in Asian countries, such as Thailand, India and Mexico, where their diet contains high levels of capsaicin, relative to western nations [21]. However, it must be remembered that these statistics only provide indirect evidence since randomized placebo controlled trials investigating the correlation of dietary capsaicin with cancer incidence have yet to be done.

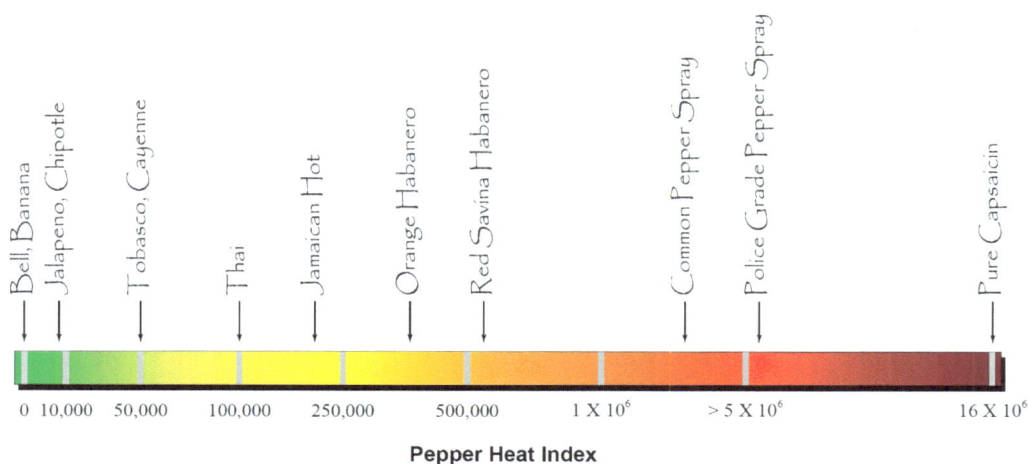

Pepper Heat Index

Figure 2: The Scoville Scale indicating the "degree of hotness" for various types of chili peppers, with pure capsaicin at the maximum parts per million. Each Scoville Unit measures 1/15 ppm of capsaicin in a chili pepper.

The biological activity of capsaicin is mediated by TRPV1 (Transient Receptor Potential subfamily Vanilloid member 1) receptor, which belongs to the TRP (Transient Receptor Potential) superfamily of cation-channel receptors [17, 18]. The TRPV receptor family is comprised of six members (TRPV1-6). Capsaicin functions as an agonist of the TRPV1 receptor. Although it is established that TRPV1 mediates the biological activity of capsaicin [16], several studies have indicated the existence of TRPV1-independent mechanisms for capsaicin action [4, 7, 22]. Many review articles have discussed the chemopreventive potential of capsaicin [2, 23, 24]; however, only a few have summarized its applications as an anti-cancer nutritional agent.

Table 1: Capsaicin dosages and administration methods used by other investigators

Dosage	Administration Route	Administration Frequency	Total Time of Experiment	Animal Model	Reference
5 mg/kg/day	Oral Gavage	3 Times/Week	3 Weeks	Nude Mice	[8]
5 mg/kg/day	Subcutaneous	3 Times/Week	2 Weeks	Nude Mice	[9]
5 mg/kg	Intragastric	Once	21 Weeks	A/J Mice	[66]
10 mg/kg	Intraperitonial	Once	16 Weeks	Swiss Albino Mice	[10]
100 mg/kg food	Diet	Continuous Feed	20 Weeks	F344 Rats	[15]
500 mg/kg food	Diet	Continuous Feed	10 Weeks	F344 Rats	[13]

The present review fills this void of knowledge and discusses the potential applications of capsaicin in the treatment of human cancers. Specifically, the growth-inhibitory activity of capsaicin in both tissue culture and animal models will be discussed. The present article also summarizes the signaling mechanisms underlying the anti-neoplastic activity of capsaicin. We believe that this detailed discussion of the anti-cancer activity of capsaicin is both timely and relevant, and will enhance our understanding of the role of nutritional agents in the therapy and management of human cancers.

Anti-neoplastic Activity of Capsaicin

Capsaicin has been shown to exhibit chemopreventive effects in animal models by suppressing carcinogenesis of the skin, colon, lung, tongue, and prostate. However, recent studies have revealed that, apart from its chemopreventive effects, capsaicin also exerts anti-cancer activity. The reader is referred to several excellent reviews that discuss the chemopreventive activity of capsaicin [2, 23-25]. The present article will focus on the anti-neoplastic activity of capsaicin in multiple types of human cancer.

Breast Cancer

Capsaicin suppressed the growth of four human breast cancer cell lines, namely BT-474, SKBR-3, MCF-7 and MDA-MB231, in a dose-and time-dependent manner. The administration of capsaicin through oral gavage reduced the volume of MDA-MB231 tumors growing orthotopically in BMX nude mice [22]. Additionally, capsaicin potently inhibited the growth of pre-neoplastic breast tumors, without any evidence of gross toxicity. In contrast, studies have also shown that the administration of capsaicin can promote mammary metastasis to the lung and heart. However, the doses of capsaicin used in latter studies were 150 mg/kg capsaicin, a pharmacological concentration aimed to produce inactivation of neurons. The study explored how this neuronal silencing contributed to the progression of mammary tumors [20].

Furthermore, these aforementioned effects of capsaicin are not specific to breast cancer cells. Studies by Oh *et al.* (2010) show that capsaicin induces cell death in MCF-10A normal human breast epithelial cells [26]. However, it must be remembered that the MCF-10A cell line is an immortalized breast epithelial cell line and has variations from normal breast epithelial cells, such as loss of the p16 locus [27].

Prostate Cancer

The nutritional agent capsaicin was found to display potent growth-inhibitory activity in both androgen-dependent and androgen-independent prostate cancers. Subcutaneous injection of capsaicin at a dose of 5 mg/kg body weight suppressed the growth of PC-3 tumors in nude mice models. The growth-inhibitory effects of capsaicin in androgen-independent PC-3 cells were mediated *via* its cognate cell surface receptor TRPV1 [9, 28, 29]. In contrast, studies by Mori *et al.* (2006) found that the growth-suppressive effects of capsaicin in PC-3 and androgen–dependent DU145 and LNCaP prostate cancer cells were mediated *via* a TRPV1-independent mechanism [8]. Additionally, data from Malagarie-Cazenave *et al.* (2009) claim that capsaicin has mitogenic effects on LNCaP cells *via* the upregulation of androgen receptor levels [30]. Such discrepancies emphasize the need for further in-depth studies to delineate precisely the molecular mechanisms underlying the growth-suppressive effects of capsaicin in human prostate cancer cells. A clinical case report by Jankovic *et al.* (2010) has shown that administration of capsaicin slowed the PSA (Prostate Specific Antigen)-doubling time in a patient with prostate cancer [31].

Lung Cancer

The treatment of lung cancer cells with capsaicin was found to trigger apoptosis in H460 human non-small cell lung cancer (NSCLC) cells [4]. Capsaicin-induced apoptosis was found to occur *via* a TRPV1-independent pathway. Capsaicin also caused cell cycle arrest in human small cell lung cancer (SCLC) cells but had no effect in normal lung epithelial cells [32]. Brown *et al.* 2010 also demonstrated the anti-proliferative activity of capsaicin in four human SCLC cell lines *in vitro* as well as in H69 SCLC tumors implanted on chicken chorioallantoic membranes (CAMs). Most interestingly, they observed that capsaicin inhibited the growth of established H69 tumors in nude mice models [32].

Colon Cancer

Capsaicin and its analog, dihydrocapsaicin (DHC), caused cell death in human HCT116 colon cancer cells [33]. DHC showed greater apoptotic activity than capsaicin in colon cancer cells [33]. Capsaicin-induced apoptosis was found to be independent of p53 status in human colon cancer cells. This is a highly significant observation since p53 is mutated in 40-50% of colorectal carcinomas, and p53 mutations are associated with aggressive colon carcinomas. Since capsaicin-induced apoptosis is independent of p53, it may be effective for the therapy and management of a large spectrum of colon cancers. Capsaicin also produces changes in cell morphology, DNA fragmentation and apoptosis in HT-29, Colo320 and LoVo human colon carcinoma cells [33-37]. Lu *et al.* (2010) have shown that capsaicin causes apoptosis in Colo205 human colon carcinoma cells xenografted in nude mice by activation of caspase-3,-8 and-9 [38].

Other Cancers

Capsaicin has been shown to cause robust apoptosis in human gastric cancer cells. It also suppresses the growth of normal gastric epithelial cells, but displays greater apoptotic activity in cancer cells [39]. Similarly, capsaicin induces cell death in human fibrosarcoma, hepatoma, glioma, melanoma, myeloma, esophageal carcinoma, pancreatic carcinoma, bladder carcinoma, tongue cancers, urothelial carcinoma and T-cell leukemia cells [3, 5, 6, 40-46]. The majority of these studies have been performed in cell culture models. It is important that these studies be extended to animal models to confirm the results obtained with human cancer cell lines. Taken together, it seems that capsaicin may be a promising anti-neoplastic agent for many different types of human cancers.

Molecular Mechanisms Underlying the Anti-neoplastic Activity of Capsaicin

Capsaicin is routinely used topically to treat pain and inflammation associated with a variety of diseases [1]. The biological activities of capsaicin are mediated by the TRPV1 (transient receptor potential cation channel subfamily vanilloid member 1) receptor, which belongs to the TRP (transient receptor potential) superfamily of cation-channel receptors [17, 18]. The TRPV receptor family is comprised of six members called TRPV1-6. Capsaicin functions as an agonist of the TRPV1 receptor [16].

A survey of existing literature shows that the growth-suppressive properties of capsaicin can either be mediated by "direct" or "indirect mechanisms". The "direct mechanisms" are a sequelae of events downstream of the binding of capsaicin to TRPV receptors on neoplastic cells (Fig. **3**). The "indirect mechanisms" are resultant of the growth-inhibitory effects of capsaicin, which are independent of the TRPV family of receptors.

Direct Mechanisms of Capsaicin

Sanchez *et al.* (2007) show that capsaicin induces apoptosis in androgen-independent PC-3 prostate cancer cells *via* TRPV1 by a mechanism involving the generation of reactive oxygen species (ROS), dissipation of mitochondrial inner transmembrane potential and activation of caspase-3 [28, 29]. In contrast, Malagarie-Cazenave *et al.* (2009) have found that capsaicin stimulates the growth of androgen-responsive LNCaP prostate cancer cells in a TRPV1-dependent manner [30]. The binding of capsaicin to TRPV1 in LNCaP cells caused increased expression of androgen receptors and activation of MAP kinase and Akt pathways, which facilitated the proliferation of LNCaP cells [30]. To further these confounding matters, Mori *et al.* (2006) have found that capsaicin causes apoptosis in LNCaP cells by a TRPV1-independent pathway [8]. Such conflicting data emphasize the need for detailed studies to examine the biological activity of capsaicin in human prostate cancer cells.

Apoptotic activity of capsaicin in glioma and urothelial cancer cells is mediated *via* the TRPV1 receptor [3, 5, 40]. RT-PCR analysis identified TRPV1 receptors in urothelial cancers, multiple glioma and glioblastoma cell lines [3, 5, 40]. Additionally, normal astrocytes were also found to express TRPV [3]. Amatini *et al.* (2007) found that the TRPV1 receptor induced the stimulation of p38 MAP kinase, which increased mitochondrial permeability and caused downstream activation of caspase-3, leading to cellular apoptosis [3]. In urothelial cancers, capsaicin caused clustering of TRPV1 receptors, stimulating activation of the Fas pathway *via* ATM kinase [40]. Capsaicin also has been found to induce degradation of the Fas associated factor FAF-1, which sensitizes cells to apoptotic cell death [40] (Fig. **3**).

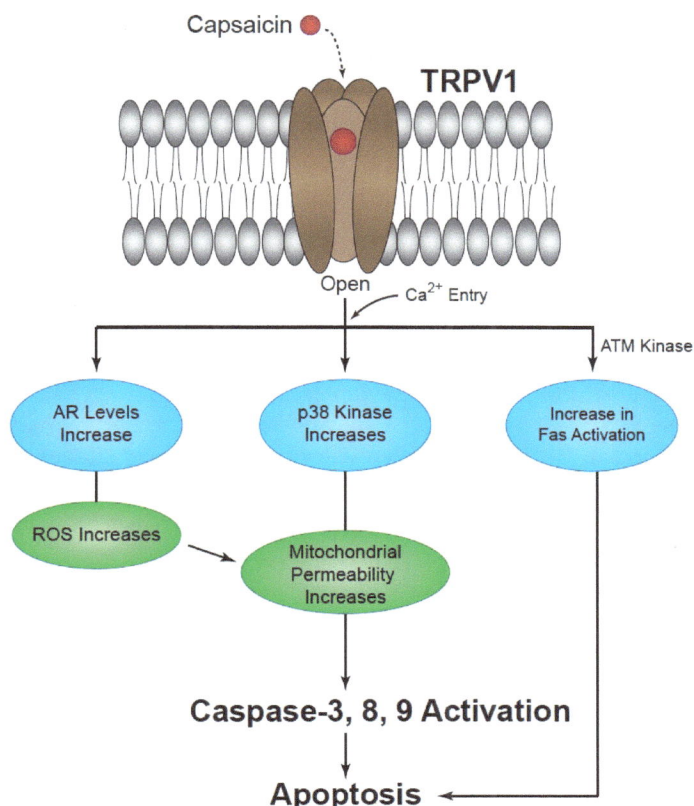

Figure 3: A schematic diagram depicting the TRPV1 receptor-dependent pathways underlying capsaicin-induced apoptosis in human cancer cells. The red dot represents capsaicin. The binding of capsaicin to the TRPV1 receptor opens the ion pore allowing the entry of calcium ions into the cell. The rise in intracellular calcium triggers multiple signaling pathways, which eventually converge upon activation of caspases and lead to cellular apoptosis.

Several studies have analyzed the differential expression of TRPV1 in normal and tumor tissues. Tissue array analysis revealed that TRPV1 gene and protein expression was inversely correlated with glioma grading, with marked loss of TRPV1 expression in grade IV glioblastoma multiforme [3]. This discovery implies that normal astrocytes have high levels of TRPV1 and cancerous glioma tissue has low TRPV1 expression. Amantini *et al.* (2007) observed that the most aggressive, advanced gliomas had very minimal or no expression of TRPV1. This result has been also observed in human urothelial cancer and lung cancer [4, 40]. Normal uroepithelial and bronchial epithelial cells have robust levels of TRPV1, whereas there is no or low expression of TRPV1 in high-grade human urothelial cancers and NSCLCs [4, 40]. Such data seems to imply that the loss of TRPV1 may be associated with the malignant transformation of tumors. If the majority of aggressive late-stage gliomas lack TRPV1, then the therapeutic potential of capsaicin as a TRPV1-agonist-based anti-cancer agent is rather unclear. However, capsaicin may have non-TRPV1 receptor-dependent effects in these tumors.

Apart from TRPV1, another member of the TRPV receptor family, namely TRPV6, has been implicated in the growth-suppressive effects of capsaicin in human gastric cancer cells [39]. TRPV6 is a cation channel receptor facilitating the entry of calcium ions into the cells in a highly selective manner. It is 100-fold more selective for calcium than sodium or potassium ions [47]. The TRPV6 receptor has been detected in tissues of the prostate, stomach, brain, intestine and lung [48]. TRPV6 is overexpressed in human prostate adenocarcinoma, whereas it is almost undetectable in benign prostate hyperplasia. The increased expression of TRPV6 correlates with tumor grade [49, 50] and clinical outcomes in prostate cancer. The fact that TRPV6 is overexpressed exclusively in tumor tissue and undetectable in normal tissue makes TRPV6 an attractive molecular target for the therapy of prostate cancer [51]. While the exact physiological function of TRPV6 in these tissues is yet to be fully understood, recent studies have speculated that TRPV6 plays a role in calcium absorption, cell proliferation, apoptosis, transepithelial calcium transport and maintenance of intracellular calcium stores in these cells [48, 52]. Studies by Chow *et al.* (2007) have shown that TRPV6 receptors mediate the apoptotic activity of capsaicin in gastric cancer cells [39] by downstream activation and stabilization of p53 as well as activation of the pro-apoptotic gene Bax. Both of these events were mediated by TRPV6-induced stimulation of the JNK pathway. A paradoxical observation is that gastric cancers do express TRPV1, yet the apoptotic actions of capsaicin are mediated by the TRPV6 receptor. Future research will need to identify the precise relationship between capsaicin and TRPV6 and, most importantly, why capsaicin utilizes the TRPV6 pathway even when TRPV1 is expressed on these gastric cancer cells.

Several convergent studies have shown that capsaicin is a ligand for the receptor TRPV1, which belongs to the TRPV superfamily of ion-channel receptors responsible for thermoregulatory functions [16]. It has been observed that capsaicin exerts apoptotic effects in certain cell lines *via* either the TRPV1 or TRPV6 receptor. In contrast, the loss of TRPV1 has been shown to correlate to oncogenesis in gliomas and human lung cancers. Such conflicting findings underscore the need for detailed studies to precisely map TRPV-dependent apoptotic pathways recruited in response to capsaicin in human cancers.

Indirect Mechanisms of Capsaicin

The anti-neoplastic activity of capsaicin is classified as being mediated by "an indirect mechanism" if it is independent of the binding of capsaicin to the TRPV family of receptors (Fig. **4**). The majority of the studies exploring the anti-cancer activity of capsaicin have implicated TRPV1-independent mechanisms for capsaicin action [4, 7]. Capsaicin has been found to suppress the growth of human cancers *via* cell cycle arrest, apoptosis or autophagy. We will discuss the mechanisms by which capsaicin induces each of these modes of growth-inhibition in multiple human cancer cell lines.

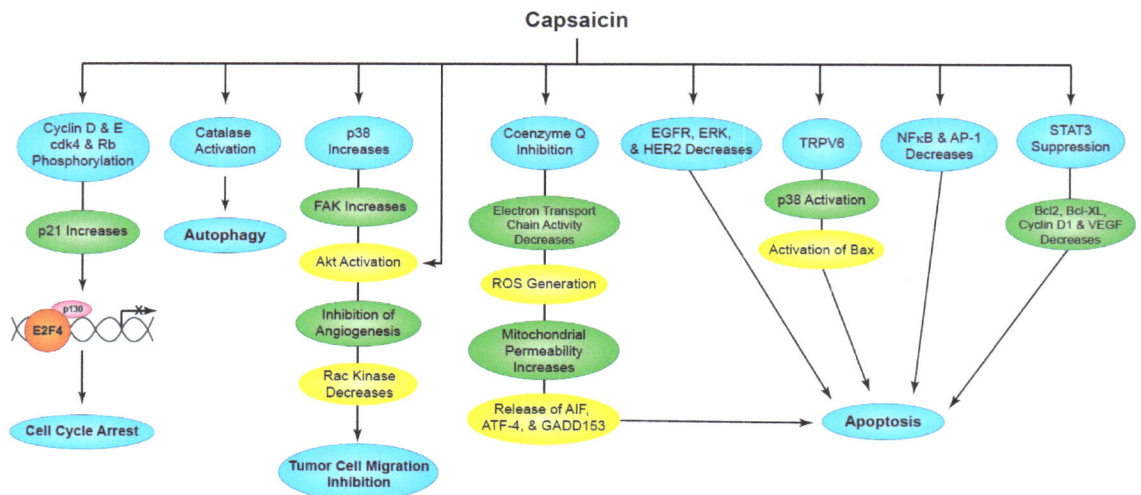

Figure 4: A representation of the non-receptor-dependent signaling pathways responsible for the anti-neoplastic activity of capsaicin in human cancer cells. Capsaicin can trigger cell cycle arrest, apoptosis and autophagy independent of TRPV receptors. In addition, capsaicin has been found to suppress angiogenesis and migration of human tumor cells by a TRPV-independent mechanism.

Cell Cycle Arrest

Capsaicin has been shown to arrest cells at the G1/S boundary *via* activation of cyclin-dependent kinase inhibitors, downregulation of cyclin D and E and cyclin-dependent kinases [53-55]. Capsaicin-induced G1 arrest in CE 81T/VGH human epidermoid carcinoma cells and prostate cancer cells occurs *via* induction of p53 and the cyclin-dependent kinase (cdk) inhibitor p21 [8, 22, 54-56]. The treatment of HL-60 human leukemic cells with capsaicin caused G1 arrest *via* inhibition of cdk2 activity [55]. The anti-angiogenic activity (discussed later in detail) of capsaicin is attributed to its ability to cause G1 arrest in endothelial cells [55]. Capsaicin-induced G1 arrest is correlated with the suppression of cyclin D1 levels, inhibition of cdk4 activity and Rb phosphorylation in endothelial and breast cancer cells [22].

Studies by Brown *et al.* (2010) demonstrated for the first time that capsaicin displayed potent anti-proliferative activity in human SCLC cell lines. Furthermore, capsaicin potently suppressed the growth of human SCLC tumors *in vivo*, as ascertained by CAM assays and nude mice models [32]. The anti-proliferative activity of capsaicin was correlated with a decrease in the expression of E2F-responsive proliferative genes, such as cyclin E, thymidylate synthase, cdc25A and cdc6, at both mRNA and protein levels. The transcription factor E2F4 was found to mediate the anti-proliferative activity of capsaicin. ChIP assays demonstrated that capsaicin caused the recruitment of E2F4 and p130 on E2F-responsive proliferative promoters, thereby inhibiting the proliferation of SCLC [32].

The majority of these studies show that the growth-inhibitory activity of capsaicin is a combination of both cell cycle arrest and apoptosis. The relative contributions of cell cycle arrest versus apoptosis in the growth-inhibitory effects of capsaicin are dependent on the nature of the cell line, the concentration of capsaicin and the duration of the treatment [54, 55]. For example, with shorter treatment periods, cell cycle arrest dominates, while apotosis contributes more to growth inhibition with longer treatment duration.

Apoptosis

Cell culture studies have investigated the signaling mechanisms underlying the apoptotic effects of capsaicin in several human cancer cell lines. The apoptotic activity of capsaicin has been found to be mediated by the upregulation of intracellular calcium in human gastric cancer, esophageal carcinoma and T-cell leukemia cells. The exact mechanism underlying the apoptotic activity of capsaicin are not yet fully understood, but the roles of NADH oxidase activity, c-Jun NH2-terminal kinase, p53 stabilization, nuclear factor-κB, activator protein-1, peroxynitrite and mitochondrial respiration have been implicated [4, 6-9, 42, 53]. An important mechanism underlying the apoptotic activity of capsaicin is the induction of ROS, which causes downstream DNA damage and cell death. Capsaicin antagonizes the function of co-enzyme Q and subsequently down regulates the activity of the electron transport chain [57]. As a result of inhibiting the electron transport chain, high amounts of ROS are delivered to the cells, causing DNA damage and apoptosis. In addition, capsaicin has also been shown to disrupt mitochondrial membrane transmembrane potential, which leads to release of pro-apoptotic proteins like AIF, ATF-4 and GADD153, leading to cell death [46].

Apart from its effects on the electron transport chain, capsaicin regulates multiple signaling pathways to induce cell death. Capsaicin is a potent inhibitor of constitutively active STAT3 and IL-6-induced STAT3 in human myeloma cells. In addition, capsaicin down regulates the levels of STAT3-responsive anti-apoptotic genes like VEGF, cyclin D1, survivin, Bcl-2 and Bcl-xL [5, 24, 42, 44, 45, 55, 58]. Thoennssissen *et al.* (2010) have demonstrated that capsaicin caused cell death in human breast cancer cells by down regulating survival pathways like ERK, EGFR and HER-2, whereas it concomitantly stimulated apoptotic signaling proteins like caspase-3 and p27 (KIP1) [22].

The treatment of gastric cancer cells, human tongue cancer cells and hepatoma cells with capsaicin has been shown to induce apoptosis *via* elevation of intracellular calcium [39, 44]. The calcium-signaling pathway controls a variety of processes, such as proliferation, gene transcription and metabolism. However, under certain conditions, the upregulation of intracellular calcium triggers apoptosis [59, 60]. The rise of intracellular calcium levels causes a decrease in Bcl-2 levels, increase in levels of Bax and downstream activation of capsases-3,-8-9, resulting in subsequent cellular apoptosis [38, 59].

Autophagy

Autophagy, or autophagocytosis, is a cell death pathway involving the degradation of a cell's own components through its lysosomal machinery [61, 62]. It is a complex, multi-step process that maintains a tightly-regulated balance between the synthesis, degradation and subsequent recycling of cellular products. Capsaicin and its analog, dihydrocapsaicin (DHC), have been found to induce autophagy in human colon and breast cancer cell lines, as well as in normal breast and lung fibroblast cells [26]. DHC induced a greater magnitude of autophagy than capsaicin [63]. Capsaicin-induced autophagy was independent of p53 status and was mediated by the activation of catalase in cells. The autophagic activity of capsaicin in normal WI38 lung fibroblasts and normal MCF-10A breast epithelial cells was regulated by the relative levels of p38, JNK and ERK activation [26, 33, 63]. Therefore, the current data suggest that capsaicin induces autophagy in cancer cells by distinctly different mechanisms relative to normal cells.

Inhibition of Angiogenesis and Migration

The effect of capsaicin on tumor angiogenesis was first investigated by Min *et al.* (2004) who found that capsaicin inhibited the proliferation of endothelial cells and displayed anti-angiogenic activity in both cell culture and mouse models [53]. Similarly, capsaicin analogs like capsiate and dihydrocapsiate have been found to inhibit VEGF-induced angiogenesis [64]. Brown *et al.* (2010) indicates that the anti-angiogenic activity of capsaicin is probably responsible, at least in part, for its observed anti-tumor activity in human SCLC as observed in nude mice and CAM models. The extent of angiogenesis observed was quantified in CAM experiments. These results showed that the capsaicin-treated H69 SCLC tumor-bearing CAM contained fewer blood vessels (3.4 ± 0.6) than those of the untreated controls (8.5 ± 0.9). The signaling mechanisms underlying the anti-angiogenic activity of capsaicin include suppression of VEGF-induced p38 mitogen-activated protein kinase, p125(FAK), and Akt activation, but its molecular target is distinct from the VEGF receptor KDR/Flk-1 [42, 53, 64].

Capsaicin has been found to suppress chemotactic motility and migration of tumor cells. The administration of capsaicin to mice blocked VEGF-induced vascular permeability and ablated the loss of vascular endothelial (VE)-cadherin-facilitated cell-cell junctions [22]. The anti-migratory effects of capsaicin in human melanoma cells were found to be due to its downregulation of the PI-3 kinase/Akt/Rac pathway [65]. The anti-angiogenic and anti-migratory activity of capsaicin may be useful not only for cancer therapy, but also for the treatment of other angiogenesis-related diseases.

CONCLUSIONS

The chemopreventive, anti-carcinogenic and anti-mutagenic effects of capsaicin have been recognized for a long time. However, recent studies have shown that capsaicin is a promising anti-cancer agent suitable for the management and treatment of multiple human cancers. Animal experiments have shown that the anti-neoplastic activity of capsaicin is achieved at low concentrations without any evidence of gross toxicity. In addition, capsaicin can also sensitize human cancer cells to TRAIL-(TNF-Related Apoptosis Inducing Ligand) induced apoptosis [57]. These findings emphasize that capsaicin may be a viable nutrition-based anti-cancer drug with applications as a single agent or in combination therapy for the treatment of a variety of human cancers.

ACKNOWLEDGEMENTS

We thank Dr. Srikumar Chellappan and his laboratory for their continuous support. The advice and suggestions of Dr. Nalini Santanam and Carla Cook are gratefully acknowledged. PDG is a recipient of a YCSA grant (82115) from the Flight Attendant Medical Research Institute, FL.

REFERENCES

[1]   Biro T, Acs G, Acs P, Modarres S, Blumberg PM. Recent advances in understanding of vanilloid receptors: a therapeutic target for treatment of pain and inflammation in skin. J Investig Dermatol Symp Proc 1997;2(1):56-60.

[2]   Aggarwal BB, Kunnumakkara AB, Harikumar KB, Tharakan ST, Sung B, Anand P. Potential of spice-derived phytochemicals for cancer prevention. Planta Med 2008;74(13):1560-9.

[3]   Amantini C, Mosca M, Nabissi M, Lucciarini R, Caprodossi S, Arcella A, *et al.* Capsaicin-induced apoptosis of glioma cells is mediated by TRPV1 vanilloid receptor and requires p38 MAPK activation. J Neurochem 2007;102(3):977-90.

[4]   Athanasiou A, Smith PA, Vakilpour S, Kumaran NM, Turner AE, Bagiokou D, *et al.* Vanilloid receptor agonists and antagonists are mitochondrial inhibitors: how vanilloids cause non-vanilloid receptor mediated cell death. Biochem Biophys Res Commun 2007;354(1):50-5.

[5]   Gil YG, Kang MK. Capsaicin induces apoptosis and terminal differentiation in human glioma A172 cells. Life Sci 2008;82(19-20):997-1003.

[6]   Hail N, Jr., Lotan R. Examining the role of mitochondrial respiration in vanilloid-induced apoptosis. J Natl Cancer Inst 2002;94(17):1281-92.

[7]   Hartel M, di Mola FF, Selvaggi F, Mascetta G, Wente MN, Felix K, *et al.* Vanilloids in pancreatic cancer: potential for chemotherapy and pain management. Gut 2006;55(4):519-28.

[8]   Mori A, Lehmann S, O'Kelly J, Kumagai T, Desmond JC, Pervan M, *et al.* Capsaicin, a component of red peppers, inhibits the growth of androgen-independent, p53 mutant prostate cancer cells. Cancer Res 2006;66(6):3222-9.

[9]   Sanchez AM, Sanchez MG, Malagarie-Cazenave S, Olea N, Diaz-Laviada I. Induction of apoptosis in prostate tumor PC-3 cells and inhibition of xenograft prostate tumor growth by the vanilloid capsaicin. Apoptosis 2006;11(1):89-99.

[10]   Anandakumar P, Kamaraj S, Jagan S, Ramakrishnan G, Vinodhkumar R, Devaki T. Stabilization of pulmonary mitochondrial enzyme system by capsaicin during benzo(a)pyrene induced experimental lung cancer. Biomed Pharmacother 2007.

[11]   Jang JJ, Kim SH, Yun TK. Inhibitory effect of capsaicin on mouse lung tumor development. *In vivo* 1989;3(1):49-53.

[12]   Park KK, Surh YJ. Effects of capsaicin on chemically-induced two-stage mouse skin carcinogenesis. Cancer Lett 1997;114(1-2):183-4.

[13]   Tanaka T, Kohno H, Sakata K, Yamada Y, Hirose Y, Sugie S, *et al.* Modifying effects of dietary capsaicin and rotenone on 4-nitroquinoline 1-oxide-induced rat tongue carcinogenesis. Carcinogenesis 2002;23(8):1361-7.

[14]   Zhang Z, Huynh H, Teel RW. Effects of orally administered capsaicin, the principal component of capsicum fruits, on the *in vitro* metabolism of the tobacco-specific nitrosamine NNK in hamster lung and liver microsomes. Anticancer Res 1997;17(2A):1093-8.

[15]   Jang JJ, Cho KJ, Lee YS, Bae JH. Different modifying responses of capsaicin in a wide-spectrum initiation model of F344 rat. J Korean Med Sci 1991;6(1):31-6.

[16]   Caterina MJ, Schumacher MA, Tominaga M, Rosen TA, Levine JD, Julius D. The capsaicin receptor: a heat-activated ion channel in the pain pathway. Nature 1997;389(6653):816-24.

[17]   Szallasi A, Blumberg PM. Vanilloid (Capsaicin) receptors and mechanisms. Pharmacol Rev 1999;51(2):159-212.

[18]   Clapham DE, Julius D, Montell C, Schultz G. International Union of Pharmacology. XLIX. Nomenclature and structure-function relationships of transient receptor potential channels. Pharmacol Rev 2005;57(4):427-50.

[19]   Conway SJ. TRPing the switch on pain: an introduction to the chemistry and biology of capsaicin and TRPV1. Chem Soc Rev 2008;37(8):1530-45.

[20]   Erin N, Zhao W, Bylander J, Chase G, Clawson G. Capsaicin-induced inactivation of sensory neurons promotes a more aggressive gene expression phenotype in breast cancer cells. Breast Cancer Res Treat 2006;99(3):351-64.

[21]   ACS. Cancer facts and figures: American Cancer Society; 2010.

[22]   Thoennissen NH, O'Kelly J, Lu D, Iwanski GB, La DT, Abbassi S, *et al.* Capsaicin causes cell-cycle arrest and apoptosis in ER-positive and-negative breast cancer cells by modulating the EGFR/HER-2 pathway. Oncogene 2010;29(2):285-96.

[23]   Oyagbemi AA, Saba AB, Azeez OI. Capsaicin: a novel chemopreventive molecule and its underlying molecular mechanisms of action. Indian J Cancer 2010;47(1):53-8.

[24]   Hail N, Jr., Lotan R. Cancer chemoprevention and mitochondria: targeting apoptosis in transformed cells *via* the disruption of mitochondrial bioenergetics/redox state. Mol Nutr Food Res 2009;53(1):49-67.

[25]   Liu EH, Qi LW, Wu Q, Peng YB, Li P. Anticancer Agents Derived from Natural Products. Mini Rev Med Chem 2009.

[26]   Oh S, Choi CH, Jung YK. Autophagy Induction by Capsaicin in Malignant Human Breast Cells is Modulated by p38 and ERK Mitogen-Activated Protein Kinases and Retards Cell Death by Suppressing Endoplasmic Reticulum Stress-Mediated Apoptosis. Mol Pharmacol 2010.

[27]   Imbalzano KM, Tartarkova I, Imbalzano AN, Nickerson JA. Increasingly transformed MCF-10A cells have a progressively tumor-like phenotype in three-dimensional basement membrane culture. Cancer Cell International 2009;9(7):1-11.

[28]   Sanchez AM, Malagarie-Cazenave S, Olea N, Vara D, Chiloeches A, Diaz-Laviada I. Apoptosis induced by capsaicin in prostate PC-3 cells involves ceramide accumulation, neutral sphingomyelinase, and JNK activation. Apoptosis 2007;12(11):2013-24.

[29]   Sanchez AM, Martinez-Botas J, Malagarie-Cazenave S, Olea N, Vara D, Lasuncion MA, *et al.* Induction of the endoplasmic reticulum stress protein GADD153/CHOP by capsaicin in prostate PC-3 cells: a microarray study. Biochem Biophys Res Commun 2008;372(4):785-91.

[30]   Malagarie-Cazenave S, Olea-Herrero N, Vara D, Diaz-Laviada I. Capsaicin, a component of red peppers, induces expression of androgen receptor *via* PI3K and MAPK pathways in prostate LNCaP cells. FEBS Lett 2009;583(1):141-7.

[31]   Jankovic B, Loblaw DA, Nam R. Capsaicin may slow PSA doubling time: case report and literature review. Can Urol Assoc J 2010;4(1):E9-E11.

[32]   Brown KC, Witte TR, Hardman WE, Luo H, Chen YC, Carpenter AB, *et al.* Capsaicin displays anti-proliferative activity against human small cell lung cancer in cell culture and nude mice models *via* the E2F pathway. PLoS One 2010;5(4):e10243.

[33]   Oh SH, Lim SC. Endoplasmic reticulum stress-mediated autophagy/apoptosis induced by capsaicin (8-methyl-N-vanillyl-6-nonenamide) and dihydrocapsaicin is regulated by the extent of c-Jun NH2-terminal kinase/extracellular signal-regulated kinase activation in WI38 lung epithelial fibroblast cells. J Pharmacol Exp Ther 2009;329(1):112-22.

[34]   Lee SH, Krisanapun C, Baek SJ. NSAID-activated gene-1 as a molecular target for capsaicin-induced apoptosis through a novel molecular mechanism involving GSK3{beta}, C/EBP{beta}, and ATF3. Carcinogenesis 2010.

[35]   Kim YM, Hwang JT, Kwak DW, Lee YK, Park OJ. Involvement of AMPK signaling cascade in capsaicin-induced apoptosis of HT-29 colon cancer cells. Ann N Y Acad Sci 2007;1095:496-503.

[36]   Kim MY, Trudel LJ, Wogan GN. Apoptosis induced by capsaicin and resveratrol in colon carcinoma cells requires nitric oxide production and caspase activation. Anticancer Res 2009;29(10):3733-40.

[37]   Yang KM, Pyo JO, Kim GY, Yu R, Han IS, Ju SA, *et al.* Capsaicin induces apoptosis by generating reactive oxygen species and disrupting mitochondrial transmembrane potential in human colon cancer cell lines. Cell Mol Biol Lett 2009;14(3):497-510.

[38]   Lu HF, Chen YL, Yang JS, Yang YY, Liu JY, Hsu SC, *et al.* Antitumor activity of capsaicin on human colon cancer cells *in vitro* and colo 205 tumor xenografts *in vivo*. J Agric Food Chem 2010;58(24):12999-123005.

[39]   Chow J, Norng M, Zhang J, Chai J. TRPV6 mediates capsaicin-induced apoptosis in gastric cancer cells--Mechanisms behind a possible new "hot" cancer treatment. Biochim Biophys Acta 2007;1773(4):565-76.

[40]   Amantini C, Ballarini P, Caprodossi S, Nabissi M, Morelli MB, Lucciarini R, *et al.* Triggering of transient receptor potential vanilloid type 1 (TRPV1) by capsaicin induces Fas/CD95-mediated apoptosis of urothelial cancer cells in an ATM-dependent manner. Carcinogenesis 2009;30(8):1320-9.

[41]   Baek YM, Hwang HJ, Kim SW, Hwang HS, Lee SH, Kim JA, *et al.* A comparative proteomic analysis for capsaicin-induced apoptosis between human hepatocarcinoma (HepG2) and human neuroblastoma (SK-N-SH) cells. Proteomics 2008;8(22):4748-67.

[42]   Bhutani M, Pathak AK, Nair AS, Kunnumakkara AB, Guha S, Sethi G, *et al.* Capsaicin is a novel blocker of constitutive and interleukin-6-inducible STAT3 activation. Clin Cancer Res 2007;13(10):3024-32.

[43]   Ghosh AK, Basu S. Fas-associated factor 1 is a negative regulator in capsaicin induced cancer cell apoptosis. Cancer Lett 2010;287(2):142-9.

[44]   Huang SP, Chen JC, Wu CC, Chen CT, Tang NY, Ho YT, *et al.* Capsaicin-induced apoptosis in human hepatoma HepG2 cells. Anticancer Res 2009;29(1):165-74.

[45]   Jun HS, Park T, Lee CK, Kang MK, Park MS, Kang HI, *et al.* Capsaicin induced apoptosis of B16-F10 melanoma cells through down-regulation of Bcl-2. Food Chem Toxicol 2007;45(5):708-15.

[46]   Ip SW, Lan SH, Huang AC, Yang JS, Chen YY, Huang HY, *et al.* Capsaicin induces apoptosis in SCC-4 human tongue cancer cells through mitochondria-dependent and-independent pathways. Environ Toxicol 2010.

[47]   Bodding M, Flockerzi V. Ca2+ dependence of the Ca2+-selective TRPV6 channel. J Biol Chem 2004;279(35):36546-52.

[48]   Nijenhuis T, Hoenderop JG, van der Kemp AW, Bindels RJ. Localization and regulation of the epithelial Ca2+ channel TRPV6 in the kidney. J Am Soc Nephrol 2003;14(11):2731-40.

[49]   Fixemer T, Wissenbach U, Flockerzi V, Bonkhoff H. Expression of the Ca2+-selective cation channel TRPV6 in human prostate cancer: a novel prognostic marker for tumor progression. Oncogene 2003;22(49):7858-61.

[50]   Wissenbach U, Niemeyer B, Himmerkus N, Fixemer T, Bonkhoff H, Flockerzi V. TRPV6 and prostate cancer: cancer growth beyond the prostate correlates with increased TRPV6 Ca2+ channel expression. Biochem Biophys Res Commun 2004;322(4):1359-63.

[51]   Wissenbach U, Niemeyer BA, Flockerzi V. TRP channels as potential drug targets. Biol Cell 2004;96(1):47-54.

[52]   Nilius B, Voets T. TRP channels: a TR(I)P through a world of multifunctional cation channels. Pflugers Arch 2005;451(1):1-10.

[53]   Min JK, Han KY, Kim EC, Kim YM, Lee SW, Kim OH, *et al.* Capsaicin inhibits *in vitro* and *in vivo* angiogenesis. Cancer Res 2004;64(2):644-51.

[54]   Wu CC, Lin JP, Yang JS, Chou ST, Chen SC, Lin YT, *et al.* Capsaicin induced cell cycle arrest and apoptosis in human esophagus epidermoid carcinoma CE 81T/VGH cells through the elevation of intracellular reactive oxygen species and Ca2+ productions and caspase-3 activation. Mutat Res 2006;601(1-2):71-82.

[55]   Tsou MF, Lu HF, Chen SC, Wu LT, Chen YS, Kuo HM, *et al.* Involvement of Bax, Bcl-2, Ca2+ and caspase-3 in capsaicin-induced apoptosis of human leukemia HL-60 cells. Anticancer Res 2006;26(3A):1965-71.

[56]   Lehen'kyi V, Flourakis M, Skryma R, Prevarskaya N. TRPV6 channel controls prostate cancer cell proliferation *via* Ca(2+)/NFAT-dependent pathways. Oncogene 2007;26(52):7380-5.

[57]   Ziglioli F, Frattini A, Maestroni U, Dinale F, Ciufifeda M, Cortellini P. Vanilloid-mediated apoptosis in prostate cancer cells through a TRPV-1 dependent and a TRPV-1-independent mechanism. Acta Biomed 2009;80(1):13-20.

[58]   Zhang R, Humphreys I, Sahu RP, Shi Y, Srivastava SK. *In vitro* and *in vivo* induction of apoptosis by capsaicin in pancreatic cancer cells is mediated through ROS generation and mitochondrial death pathway. Apoptosis 2008;13(12):1465-78.

[59]   Roderick HL, Cook SJ. Ca2+ signalling checkpoints in cancer: remodelling Ca2+ for cancer cell proliferation and survival. Nat Rev Cancer 2008;8(5):361-75.

[60]   Munaron L, Antoniotti S, Lovisolo D. Intracellular calcium signals and control of cell proliferation: how many mechanisms? J Cell Mol Med 2004;8(2):161-8.

[61]   Barth S, Glick D, Macleod KF. Autophagy: assays and artifacts. J Pathol 2010;221(2):117-24.

[62]   Glick D, Barth S, Macleod KF. Autophagy: cellular and molecular mechanisms. J Pathol 2010;221(1):3-12.

[63]   Oh SH, Kim YS, Lim SC, Hou YF, Chang IY, You HJ. Dihydrocapsaicin (DHC), a saturated structural analog of capsaicin, induces autophagy in human cancer cells in a catalase-regulated manner. Autophagy 2008;4(8):1009-19.

[64]   Pyun BJ, Choi S, Lee Y, Kim TW, Min JK, Kim Y, *et al.* Capsiate, a nonpungent capsaicin-like compound, inhibits angiogenesis and vascular permeability *via* a direct inhibition of Src kinase activity. Cancer Res 2008;68(1):227-35.

[65]   Shin DH, Kim OH, Jun HS, Kang MK. Inhibitory effect of capsaicin on B16-F10 melanoma cell migration *via* the phosphatidylinositol 3-kinase/Akt/Rac1 signal pathway. Exp Mol Med 2008;40(5):486-94.

[66]   Teel RW , Huynh HT. Lack of inhibitory effect of intragastically administered capsaicin on NNK-induced lung tumor formation in the A.J. mouse. *In vivo* 1999;(13):231-234.

CHAPTER 3

Omega-3 Fatty Acids as an Adjuvant to Cancer Therapy

Elaine W. Hardman[*]

Nutrition and Cancer Center and Departments of Biochemistry and Microbiology, Joan C. Edwards School of Medicine, Marshall University, Huntington, WV, USA

Abstract: The growth of various types of cancers including lung, colon, mammary, and prostate in animal models has been slowed by supplementing the diet of the tumor-bearing mice or rats with oils containing omega-3 (n-3) fatty acids or with purified n-3 fatty acids. The efficacy of cancer chemotherapy drugs such as doxorubicin, epirubicin, CPT-11, 5-fluorouracil, and tamoxifen and of radiation therapy has been improved when the diet included n-3 fatty acids. A number of potential mechanisms have been identified for the activity of n-3 fatty acids against cancer including modulation of: eicosanoid production and inflammation, angiogenesis, proliferation, susceptibility for apoptosis, estrogen signaling and free radical activity. The response to chemotherapy was better in breast cancer patients with higher levels of n-3 fatty acids in adipose tissue (indicating past consumption of n-3 fatty acids) than in patients with lower levels of n-3 fatty acids in one study. Omega-3 fatty acids have also been used to suppress cancer-associated cachexia and improve the quality of life in human studies. Thus, supplementing the diet with n-3 fatty acids may be a nontoxic means to improve the outcome of standard cancer therapies and may slow or prevent recurrence of cancer in patients that are not candidates for standard cancer treatments.

Keywords: Arachidonic Acid, Cancer, Corn Oil, Cyclooxygenase, Docosahexaenoic Acid, Diet, Eicosanoid, Eicosapentaenoic Acid, Fatty Acid, Fish, Fish Oil, Food, Nutrition, PPAR-Gamma.

INTRODUCTION

The growth of chemically induced cancers and of human cancer xenografts in animal models has been slowed or completely inhibited by incorporation of omega 3 (n-3) fatty acids in the diet of the host mouse or rat (examples: [1-5]). The results of the few reported human studies also indicate that omega 3 fatty acids may improve the outcome of cancer therapy [6] or improve the quality of life if consumed prior to or during human cancer therapy [7]. The objective of this chapter is to briefly review the evidence for the benefits of omega-3 fatty acids on cancer growth or cancer therapy and to present rational mechanisms for those effects. Increased interest in nontoxic alternative therapies for cancer and the development of new molecular biology techniques are rapidly expanding our knowledge of mechanisms for the effects of omega 3 fatty acids on cancer growth.

WHAT ARE OMEGA-3 FATTY ACIDS?

Fatty acids are hydrocarbon chains with a carboxyl group at the head (delta) end and a methyl group at the tail (n or omega) end (Fig. **1**). The carbons in the chain may be connected by single or double bonds. The number of carbons in the chain and the type of bond between the carbons gives rise to the different types of fatty acids. In saturated fatty acids, the bonds between all carbons are single bonds and are fully saturated with hydrogen. Mono-and polyunsaturated fatty acids have one or more double bonds connecting some carbons thus these bonds are not saturated with hydrogen. The first double bond in an omega 6 (n-6) fatty acid is 6 carbons from the 'n' end; the first double bond in an omega 3 fatty acid is 3 carbons from the 'n' end. Humans and other mammals can synthesize saturated fatty acids and monounsaturated (n-9) fatty acids but cannot desaturate either the n-6 or the n-3 double bond. N-3 and n-6 fatty acids are essential components in cell membrane phospholipids and as a substrate for enzymes that synthesize various molecules. Thus, it is essential to consume n-3 and n-6 fatty acids in the diet.

*Address Correspondence to Elaine W. Hardman: Nutrition and Cancer Center, Department of Biochemistry and Microbiology, Joan C. Edwards School of Medicine, Marshall University, Byrd Biotechnology Science Center, Room 336S, 1700 Third Avenue, Huntington WV, 25755, USA; E-mail: hardmanw@marshall.edu

Pier Paolo Claudio and Richard M. Niles (Eds)

Eighteen carbon n-3 and n-6 fatty acids are available from plant sources. N-6 fatty acid is consumed primarily as linoleic acid (abbreviated as 18:2n6 meaning 18 carbons, 2 double bonds, n-6 type) from vegetable oils (corn, peanut, soybean) and vegetables, but some arachidonic acid (AA, 20:4n-6) is also obtained from meats [8]. N-3 fatty acids may be consumed as α-linolenic acid (18:3n-3), which is contained in various amounts in some oils (canola (11% 18:3n-3), flaxseed (57%), soybean (8%)) and in leafy green vegetables. Longer-chain n-3 fatty acids, mainly eicosapentaenoic (EPA, 20:5n-3) and docosahexaenoic (DHA, 22:6n-3) acids, are found in fish and fish oils. N-3 and n-6 fatty acids cannot be interconverted but both can be elongated and desaturated to form other fatty acids of the same series [9]. Humans have the enzymes to elongate and desaturate 18:3n-3 to EPA and DHA but it is not clear how important this pathway for the formation of EPA and DHA is in humans. Certainly a good source of EPA and DHA is from fish or fish oils in the diet. The activity of Δ5 and Δ6 desaturases, essential for the production of AA from linoleic acid, is suppressed by the 3 major n-3 fatty acids, α-linolenic acid, EPA, and DHA [10].

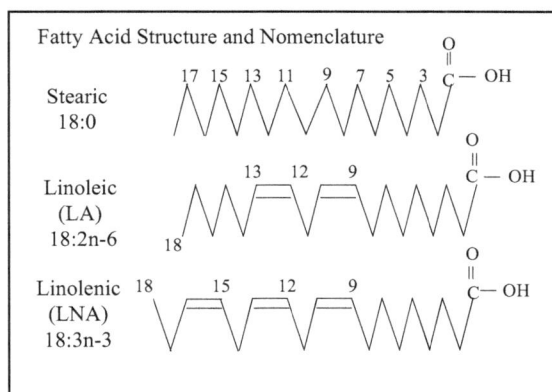

Figure 1: Structures of fatty acids. Stearic acid is an 18-carbon saturated fat. Linoleic acid is an 18-carbon fatty acid with 2 unsaturated bonds and with an unsaturation in the n-6 position, thus the abbreviation is 18:2n-6. Alpha-linolenic acid is an 18-carbon n-3 fatty acid with 3 double bonds.

WHY IS REDUCTION OF AA CONTENT IMPORTANT?

Cyclooxygenase (COX) and lipoxygenase (LOX) act on 20-carbon fatty acids (either AA or EPA) to produce cell signaling molecules. COX activity on AA or EPA produces prostaglandins or thromboxanes; LOX activity on AA or EPA produces leukotrienes, hydroxy fatty acids and epoxy fatty acids. Suppression of AA production by n-3 fatty acids reduces the substrate available for the production of the AA-derived eicosanoids. Eicosanoids made from AA, including prostaglandin E_2, thromboxane A_2, leukotriene B_4, and 12-hydroxyeicosatetraenoic acid, tend to promote inflammation and proliferation in most tissues and have been shown to be promotional to carcinogenesis [11]. In contrast, the eicosanoids produced from EPA, prostaglandin E_3 and leukotriene B_5, are produced less efficiently (PGE_3) or are far less promotional to inflammation (PGE_3 and LTB_5) than AA derived eicosanoids; thus, EPA-derived eicosanoids are less favorable for the development and growth of cancer cells.

EFFECTS OF N-3 ON EICOSANOID SYNTHESIS

COX has 2 isozymes: COX 1 and COX 2. COX 1 is constitutively produced by most cell types and COX 2 is produced as part of the inflammatory response. Because inflammation has been associated with cancer promotion, the use of COX inhibitors to reduce inflammation has shown promise as a cancer preventive strategy [12-14]. Incorporation of n-3 fatty acids in the diet can reduce the inflammatory response in multiple ways. These mechanisms include: 1) EPA has been shown to suppress the production of COX 2 [15, 16] thus suppressing the synthesis of prostanoids; 2) the presence of EPA in the membrane makes EPA available as a substrate for the COX that is produced thus changing the type of prostanoid that is synthesized and suppressing the inflammatory response [17]; 3) n-3 polyunsaturated fatty acids increase the catabolism of eicosanoids [18] and 4) EPA out-competes AA for COX and LOX [19-21]. The eicosanoids derived from n-3 fatty acids can also inhibit the production of AA derived eicosanoids. In fact, EPA derived 15-hydroperoxyeicosapentaenoic acid is even more inhibitory to the synthesis of eicosanoids from AA then is EPA [22].

EFFECTS OF N-3 FATTY ACIDS ON CANCER AND THE HOST

Supplementing the diet of tumor-bearing mice or rats with oils containing EPA or DHA has slowed the growth of various types of cancers including lung [23, 24], colon [25, 26], mammary [27-29], and prostate [30].

Our data (Fig. **2** from [32]) will be used to illustrate the profound growth suppression of a small amount of dietary n-3 fatty acids on a human breast cancer xenograft. This figure illustrates the mean growth rate of MDA-MB 231 xenografts in nude mice that were consuming either a diet containing 5% w/w corn oil (corn oil is 50% n-6 fatty acid) or 2% w/w corn oil + 3% w/w of an n-3 fatty acid product containing ~63% n-3 fatty acids (Incell AAFA™). Nude mice consuming an AIN 76 semipurified diet were implanted subcutaneously with ~10^6 MDA-MB 231 human breast cancer cells. After the tumors were ~5 mm in diameter, the diets of groups of tumor-bearing mice (n = 10 per group) were changed to the experimental diets. The mean tumor size of each group was not different at the time of diet change. This experimental design assures that the effects on tumor growth are not due to differences in tumor cell 'take' but to the effect of the diet on tumor growth. It is expected that any dietary effects would not be evident until after adequate n-3 fatty acid has been incorporated into tumor cell phospholipids thus the data on the graph starts at day 14 after dietary change, the mean tumor size at each time is shown. Even 14 days after diet change it appears that the n-3 supplemented diet is beginning to effect tumor growth. Linear regression analysis using the individual data from each mouse was used to determine the tumor growth rates; t-tests of the tumor growth rates showed that the growth rate of the tumors of mice fed the diet containing n-3 fatty acid was significantly less than the growth rate of the tumors of mice fed the corn oil diet (p < 0.05).

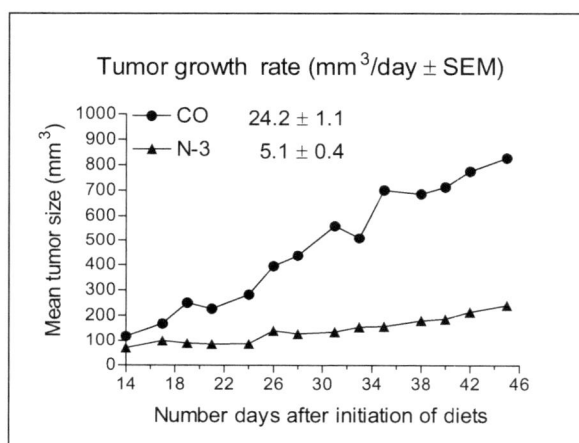

Figure 2: Growth rates of MDA-MB 231 tumors in mice fed diets containing 5% w/w corn oil or 2% w/w corn oil and 3% w/w n-3 enriched AAFA.

N-3 fatty acids have been shown to increase the efficacy of various cancer chemotherapy drugs and of radiation therapy against cancer. For example, the efficacies of doxorubin, [23, 32, 33], epirubicin [34], 5-fluorouracil [35], mitomycin C [36], arabinosylcytosine [37], tamoxifen [38], and CPT-11 [28, 35] and of radiation therapy [39] have been enhanced when long-chain n-3 fatty acids were included in the diet of animals or culture medium of cells being treated.

Again, our data (Fig. **3**, from [32]) will be used to illustrate the enhancement of the efficacy of a chemotherapy when n-3 fatty acids are included in the diet. This graph shows two additional groups of mice of the experiment described above. After two weeks of consumption of the diets, mice from each dietary group were randomly selected for initiation of doxorubicin (DOX) therapy. Doxorubicin was administered at 5 mg/kg body weight each 4 days, i.v. in a lateral tail vein. After two weeks of DOX treatment, mice were losing excess weight at this schedule of DOX treatment so the spacing of injections was increased to each seven days for the next three weeks and mouse weight stabilized. Thus if day 0 was the day of the first injection, mice received DOX injections on days 0, 4, 8, 12, 19, 26, and 33 and were sacrificed on day 34. As can be seen from the data on the graph, DOX did suppress tumor growth in mice that were consuming the n-6 (corn oil) diet. However, tumor growth suppression was not significantly better than consumption of the n-3 diet enriched alone. Addition of DOX treatment to mice that consumed the n-3 diet resulted in an additional significant suppression of tumor growth, in fact, tumor growth was stopped for the remainder of the experiment.

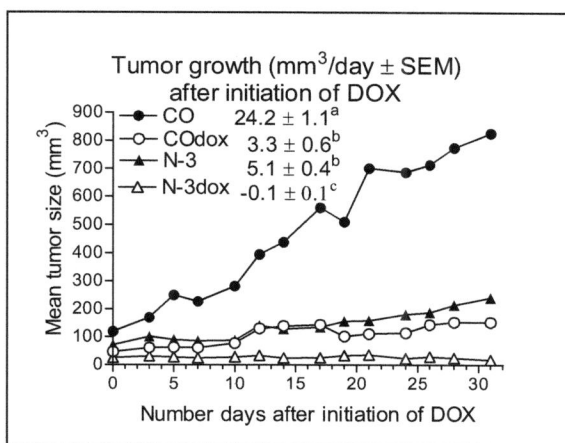

Figure 3: Growth rates of MDA-MB 231 tumors in mice fed diets containing 5% w/w corn oil or 2% w/w corn oil and 3% w/w n-3 enriched AAFA with and without doxorubicin treatment. Growth rates with different superscripts are significantly different.

Consumption of n-3 fatty acids may also reduce cancer cachexia. Cachexia is the wasting away of lean mass that is not corrected by increasing caloric consumption. Pancreatic cancer patients often develop debilitating cachexia. Some have shown weight gain and improved quality of life after daily supplementation of the diet with a calorie and protein dense (610 kcal, 32.2 g protein) liquid supplement containing 2.2g EPA and 0.96 g DHA [41]. Patients who consumed the supplement that contained calories and protein but that did not contain the n-3 fatty acids did not gain weight.

We, and others, have also shown that the side effects of cancer chemotherapies may be reduced by supplementing the diet with n-3 fatty acids. For example, irinotecan (CPT-11) is a camptothecin derivative that has shown good efficacy against colon cancer [42] and is beginning to be used against breast cancer. However, people cannot tolerate CPT-11 for very long due to the massive diarrhea resulting from intestinal damage. The CPT-11 specific diarrhea is associated with increased production of thromboxane A_2 and increased inflammation in the intestine [43-45]. Mice do not develop diarrhea following CPT-11 treatment but the intestinal mucosal damage seen following CPT-11 treatment is similar to that seen in human intestine following CPT-11 treatment [46]. Since the damage is mediated by thromboxane A_2 and prostaglandin E_2, suppression of these AA derived prostanoid production might result in decreased damage [45]. As shown in Fig. **4** [28] intestinal damage was ameliorated by a diet containing 3% fish oil.

From another report, supplementing the diet of CPT-11 treated mice with only 2% w/w of n-3 rich AAFA™: decreased apoptotic figures in the duodenal crypts; markedly suppressed the inflammatory eicosanoid, prostaglandin E_2 (PGE$_2$) in the liver; prevented liver hypertrophy; improved white blood cell counts; significantly increased red blood cell (RBC) counts; and restored grooming behavior [40]. Eighty three percent of humans also report asthenia (tiredness or weakness) as a side effect of CPT-11 treatment [47]. In mice, asthenia could be demonstrated by behavioral changes such as lack of grooming. Grooming behavior was maintained in mice that consumed the n-3 enriched diet [40] a behavior that might translate to less asthenia in humans.

The fish oil containing diet also increased the efficacy of the CPT-11 [28]. The reduction of the detrimental side effects as well as the increase in efficacy of the chemotherapy could allow for longer term treatment and potentially a better outcome for patients.

MECHANISMS FOR THE EFFECTS OF N-3 FATTY ACIDS AGAINST CANCER

Multiple mechanisms have been proposed for suppression of tumor cell growth by n-3 fatty acids. The results of experiments using new molecular biology techniques are providing additional knowledge of the regulation of gene expression by fatty acids. It is likely that suppression of tumor cell growth by n-3 fatty acids is due to the combination of these mechanisms rather than to a single, unique activity that is THE sole mechanism of action. Some of the mechanisms proposed for the action of n-3 fatty acids against cancer are as follows:

Effects of CPT-11 and omega 3 fatty acids on colon morphology

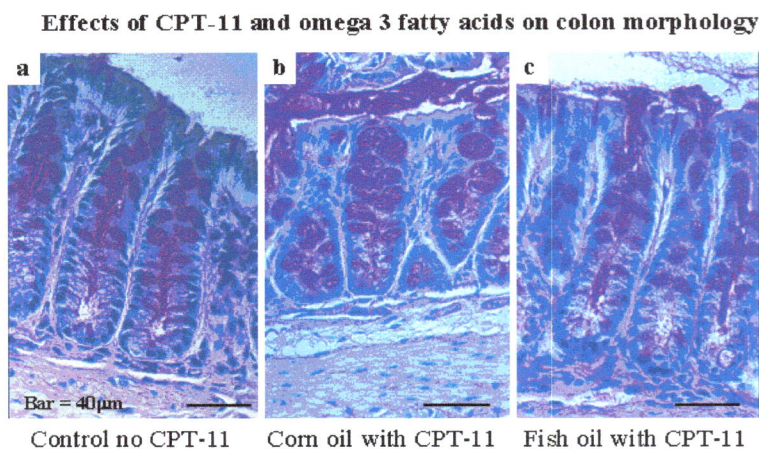

Control no CPT-11   Corn oil with CPT-11   Fish oil with CPT-11

Figure 4: Large intestinal morphology of mice fed diets containing 7% corn oil or 4% corn oil and 3% fish oil. A dose of 60 mg CPT-11/kg body weight (about 0.08 ml/28 g mouse) was injected into the lateral tail vein of each treated mouse, once each 4 days for 2 weeks. Mice were killed 24 hours after the last CPT-11 treatment. A one cm segment of each large intestine located 4cm from the anus was removed, open and placed flat on card stock for formalin fixation. Paraffin blocked sections were stained by the periodic acid-Schiff (PAS) reaction and counterstained with hematoxylin to identify mucin in goblet cells. In the colon of CPT-11 treated mice fed 7% corn oil, the muscularis mucosa was significantly thinner and the mean crypt column height was significantly shorter than in the colon of mice not treated with CPT-11. The shorter column height was accompanied by a significant increase in number of goblet cells. A diet which included 3% fish oil prevented CPT-11-induced goblet cell hyperplasia in the colon and the intestinal mucosal architecture of these mice was largely the same as the intestinal mucosal architecture of the mice not treated with CPT-11. From [40].

If n-3 fatty acids are available, they will be used as a substrate by COX 2. It has been reported that DHA inhibits eicosanoid synthesis from AA [48], EPA is preferred over AA as a substrate for COX [49], and that EPA out-competes AA for COX activity [17, 49]. The result is that if n-3 fatty acids are included in the diet and made available in cellular phospholipids, less of the inflammation-producing and growth-promoting prostaglandin E_2 will be produced in normal and in tumor tissues. Since prostaglandin E_2 feeds back to increase activation of COX, reduction in prostaglandin E_2 production helps to reduce the activity of COX.

Many tumor types overexpress COX 2 [50] and tumor growth can be slowed by COX 2 inhibitors such as celecoxib [51, 52]. As shown in Fig. **5** [31], whether by direct or indirect mechanisms, consumption of n-3 fatty acids suppresses COX 2.

Residual and metastatic tumor cells must multiply for the tumor to recur or for metastatic cells to grow into a life-threatening tumor. AA promotes growth by activating protein kinase C to stimulate mitosis [53]; n-3 fatty acids do not activate protein kinase C. ras and AP1 are transcription factors for many growth-promoting genes; N-3 fatty acids have been shown to decrease the activation of oncogenic ras and AP1 [54, 55]. The AA-derived products of COX and LOX stimulate mitosis whereas the EPA-derived products of COX and LOX decrease cancer growth [56, 57]. Thus n-3 fatty acids can slow growth of cancer cells by direct action on transcription factors and by the second messenger activity of products of EPA metabolism.

When activated, the transcription factor, nuclear factor κB (NFκB), blocks programmed cell death or apoptosis [58]. NFκB is often activated at high levels in cancer cells, resulting in cells that do not die in response to the genetic damage and that are resistant to chemotherapy drugs or radiation. N-3 fatty acids can restore functional apoptosis by downregulating NFκB [58] and can restore the sensitivity of the cancer to chemotherapy. Our data in Fig. **6** [31] illustrates the suppression of the activation of NFκB by consumption of n-3 fatty acids. Since NFκB is a transcription factor for COX 2, suppression of the activity of NFκB also downregulates COX 2 expression [59, 60] and effects COX related tumor promotion.

The Bcl-2 family of genes can also block apoptosis, resulting in cells that do not die at the appropriate time. Omega 3 fatty acids can increase response to chemotherapy and slow growth of cancer cells by downregulating the expression of Bcl-2 family genes [61, 62].

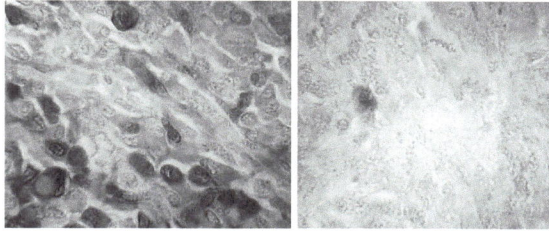

Figure 5: Suppression of cyclooxygenase (COX) 2 expression by n-3 fatty acids: Immunohistochemical localization of COX 2 (dark stain) in MDA-MB 231 xenografts grown in nude mice. Upper panel: a tumor from a mouse fed a diet containing 5% by weight (w/w) corn oil, the bottom frame; Lower panel: a tumor from a mouse fed a diet containing 2% w/w corn oil and 3% w/w of an n-3 fatty acid product containing ~63% n-3 fatty acids. Consumption of n-3 fatty acid markedly suppressed COX 2 expression. From [31].

Terminally differentiated cells do not proliferate. Cancer cells are typically less differentiated that the normal counterparts, so induction of differentiation in could stop the growth of tumors. N-3 fatty acids have been shown to suppress proliferation and induce terminal differentiation in breast cancer cells [63].

New blood vessels must develop as cancers grow to supply nutrients to the cells and to remove wastes. Suppression of angiogenesis has been proposed as a strategy to prevent or limit tumor growth [64]. Both PGE_2 and COX 2 have been shown to be promotional to angiogenesis [65-67]. N-3 fatty acids can inhibit angiogenesis by altering prostaglandin production and by inhibition of protein kinase C [66]. N-3 fatty acids have also reduced tumor growth by inhibition of vascular endothelial growth factor (VEGF) [68] and by suppression of tube forming activity [69] an early step in the formation of new blood vessels. Since VEGF may protect endothelial cells from irradiation induced apoptosis [70], reducing VEGF expression may be help restore tumor sensitivity to radiation therapy.

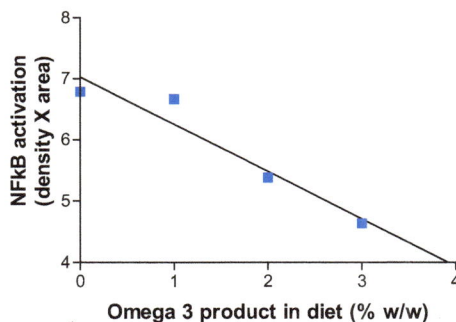

Figure 6: Suppression of the activation of nuclear factor κB (NFκB) by n-3 fatty acids. NFκB in the nuclear fraction is considered to be activated NFκB. This figure shows the mean results of electrophoretic mobility shift assay of NFκB in the nuclear fraction of livers of mice fed 8% w/w dietary fat. Part of the dietary fat was corn oil (8% to 5% in decreasing amounts); the remainder of the dietary fat was an n-3 fatty acid product (0 to 3% w/w in increasing amounts) containing 63% n-3 fatty acids. Equal amounts of protein were placed in each lane, $n = 2$ to 3 mice per diet. The density of the bands on the gel shift was quantified using NIH Image and NFκB was calculated as a product of the area of each band and the density of each pixel. From [31].

Many early breast cancers are estrogen dependent. Prostaglandin E_2, a product of AA, activates P450 aromatase and increases the aromatization of androstenedione to produce estrogen [71]. However, PGE_3 does not induce aromatase. Reduced PGE_2 following consumption of n-3 fatty acids could decrease estrogen stimulation of these tumors thus decreasing the growth of estrogen-dependent breast cancers. Our data (Fig. 7) indicate that plasma estrogen is reduced in female mice that consumed an omega 3 supplemented diet.

Free radical activity and enhanced oxidative stress play a promotional role in cancer initiation and growth. We have found that only 3% w/w fish oil in the diet can increase endogenous antioxidative enzyme activity in normal tissues of mice [32] and would be expected to reduce oxidative stress in these tissues. Since NFκB is responsive to oxidative stress, the decreased oxidative stress would also reduce NFκB activity.

Other potential mechanisms for n-3 activity include: suppression of ornithine decarboxylase activity, alteration in cell membrane fluidity, increasing insulin sensitivity and activation of PPARγ. Ornithine decarboxylase (ODC) is the rate limiting enzyme for polyamine synthesis and thus is involved in cell proliferation. ODC activity has been shown to be decreased in rats [72] and in humans [73] following consumption of n-3 fatty acids. Changes in cell membrane fluidity alters the functions of transmembrane proteins [74] and the ability of the cell to metastasize [75-77]. Epidemiological and experimental evidence is increasing that hyperinsulinemia is promotional to cancer and may be part of the link between cancer and obesity [78]. Increasing endogenous insulin sensitivity would be expected to decrease insulin levels and reduce promotion of proliferation. Fatty acids are natural ligands for the PPARs (peroxisome proliferator-activater receptors) [74]. Activation of PPARγ is associated with inhibition of the activities of NFkB, AP-1 and STAT transcription factors, three important transcription factors in cytokine gene expression [79].

In summary, multiple mechanisms can play a role in suppression of tumor growth by n-3 fatty acids. Some of the mechanisms may play a more dominant role in particular tumor types (*i.e.* alteration of estrogen is likely to be more important for suppression of breast cancer than for esophageal cancer). However, the proposed mechanisms are not mutually exclusive and it is likely that multiple mechanisms contribute to suppression of cancer growth.

FEASIBILITY OF USE IN HUMAN CANCER TREATMENT

The results of animal studies are quite promising that n-3 fatty acids may be a clinically useful addition to cancer therapy. However, a very high level of n-3 supplement was used in many of the animal studies, often 20–24% (by weight) of the diet. We have used a much lower amount of dietary fat in our more recent studies, 3% w/w or less of the mouse diet. Based on caloric consumption, we have estimated this to be equivalent to about 12g of an n-3 supplement in an 1800 calorie diet. If a human were to consume 12g of supplement per day, consumption of an n-3 concentrate, such as Incel AAFA™ (45% EPA and 10% DHA) would provide more of the desirable long chain fatty acids than the fish oil concentrates (18% EPA and 12% DHA) that are readily available in stores. Results of animal studies may be a useful proof of concept and can be used to investigate mechanisms of action, but it is also important to know how much n-3 fat can be consumed by humans and whether this amount can effectively suppress cancer growth.

Plasma estrogen and litter size of female mice fed 10% w/w corn oil or 5% w/w canola oil with 5% w/w omega 3 supplement. n = 5 mice/group		
	10% corn oil	5% canola/5% omega 3
Plasma estrogen	1.86 ng/ml	1.35 ng/ml
Mean litter size	7.2 pups/litter	6.8 pups/litter

Figure 7: Plasma estrogen and litter size of female mice fed n-6 or n-3 enriched diets. Our unpublished data.

Burns *et al.* reported the results of a phase 1 (dose-tolerance) trial using an n-3 supplement (about 38% EPA and 25% DHA) and in this study the maximum tolerated dose of this supplement was 0.3 g/kg per day or up to 21 g/d for a 70-kg patient [80]. It should be noted that subjects in this study were pancreatic cancer patients and that these sick cancer patients could tolerate this amount of n-3 supplement. Twenty-one capsules contained about 13.1 g of EPA plus DHA per day. A number of reports from the group of K.C. Fearon, M.J. Tisdale, S.J. Wigmore, M.D. Barber, *et al.* cite the effects of n-3 fatty acid supplements on weight loss in pancreatic cancer patients. Early studies found that weight loss was ameliorated and that the patients actually began to gain weight using as much as 12 g fish oil (18% EPA/12% DHA) per day [81]. The results of later studies indicate that 2.2 g EPA + 0.96 g DHA per day contained in a protein-and energy-dense supplement would ameliorate weight loss and improve the quality of life of pancreatic cancer patients significantly better than the supplement without EPA [41]. This group has also reported the effects of the nutritional supplement on metabolic mediators in pancreatic cancer patients [7]. In this study, serum IL-6 and excreted proteolysis-inducing factor were significantly reduced in the group that consumed EPA. The results of a study on the effects of EPA without or with megestrol acetate indicated that EPA increased appetite and weight gain in patients with cancer-associated wasting [82] but the increase was not any better than the increase due to megestrol. The patients in the later study consumed 2.18 g/d of EPA. Information gained from the 2 studies indicates that an effective dose of EPA to reduce cachexia may be between 2 and 4 g/d. Taken together, these data indicate that humans can consume enough n-3 fatty acids to influence cytokine production and that only small amounts of n-3 may be required to significantly influence cell cytokines.

A report by Bougnoux *et al.* [83] presents some evidence that n-3 fatty acids may be useful during human cancer therapy. The fatty acid composition of breast adipose tissue of breast cancer patients was determined. The results indicated that patients with complete or partial remission in response to cytotoxic drugs had a higher level of DHA in the breast adipose tissue than did patients with no response or progression following therapy. This higher level of DHA represented increased long-term consumption of n-3 fatty acids by these patients. It is also possible to increase DHA in breast tissue by short-term (3 mo) consumption of n-3 fatty acids [84] thus increasing the consumption of n-3 fatty acids prior to and during cancer therapy may be useful. Even though scant in number, these reports provide encouraging evidence that n-3 fatty acids may be beneficial for cancer therapy in humans.

It is generally thought that the ratio of n-3 to n-6 may be more important than the absolute amounts of fatty acids that are consumed [85]. This is a logical conclusion since these types of fatty acids compete for the activity of the same enzymes. In this regard, reducing the consumption of n-6 fatty acids and increasing consumption of n-3 fatty acids may be useful. One beneficial dietary change would be to increase the consumption of n-3 containing fish, especially cold water fish, and to reduce the consumption of beef and pork. Another strategy is to change consumption of vegetable fats and oils to those that contain less n-6 fatty acid. Fig. **8** is a table of the major fatty acid types found in readily available oils. It can be seen that the compositions of the fats and oils is widely varied. Saturated and monounsaturated fats are not considered to effect cancer incidence and growth either positively or negatively. However, saturated fat causes detrimental effects to the cardiovascular system so it should not be consumed in large quantities. Olive oil is a good choice as it is predominately monounsaturated fat and is very low in n-6 fat. Canola oil is also a good choice for baking and frying, when the distinctive taste of olive oil is not desired, as the n-3/n-6 ratio is 1:2 and is has the next lowest amount of n-6 fatty acids. Soybean oil also has 8% n-3 fatty acids but it contains a high percentage of n-6 fatty acids thus the n-3/n-6 ratio is not as good as with canola oil.

Dietary n-3 fatty acids are also known to slow platelet function and in this role are beneficial for prevention cardiovascular disease. They could be concern that consumption of high amounts of n-3 fatty acids might cause clinically significant bleeding problems. However, even consumption of 6 g/DHA per day did not induce statistical differences in bleeding times of healthy volunteers [86]. Consumption of n-3 fatty acids has been shown to be beneficial against heart disease for the anti-inflammatory and anti-thrombotic benefits [87].

In conclusion, preclinical studies indicate that n-3 fatty acids should be beneficial for cancer treatment; mechanistic studies indicate feasible mechanisms for the influence of n-3 fatty acids on tumor growth, survival, and response to chemotherapy; and a limited number of clinical studies indicate that n-3 fatty acids may be beneficial when consumed before chemotherapy. It seems important to commence human trials using an n-3 fatty acid as a supplement to standard chemotherapy to determine if n-3 fatty acids can increase therapeutic response and improve the quality of life of humans with cancer. The proposed mechanisms of action may also have benefit for prevention of cancer yet to date few studies have investigated the cancer preventive potential of consumption of omega 3 fatty acids.

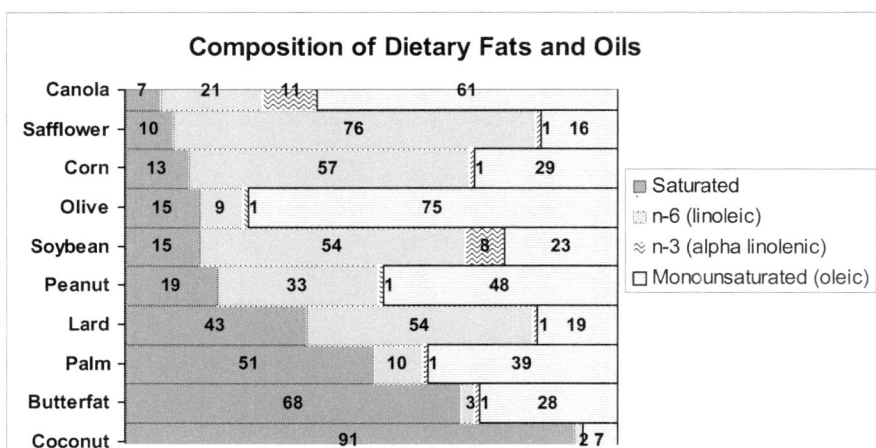

Figure 8: Comparison of the fatty acid content of dietary fats and oils. Data from POS Pilot Plant Corporation, Saskatoon, Saskatchewan, Canada, June 1994. Available from Canola Council of Canada, Publications, Fat Charts, athttp://www.canola-council.org/.

ACKNOWLEDGEMENTS

Our work has been supported through the years by grants from the American Institute for Cancer Research, the Susan G. Komen Breast Cancer Research Foundation, the National Cancer Institute and the Department of Defense Breast Cancer Research Program.

Part of the information in this chapter has been previously published in: Hardman, WE. The influence of ω-3 PUFAs on chemo-or Radiation Therapy for Cancer. In: Dietary Omega-3 Polyunsaturated Fatty Acids and Cancer. Calviello, G. and Serini, S. editors, Springer. January 2010

REFERENCES

[1]   Begin ME, Ells G, Das UN, Horrobin DF. Differential killing of human carcinoma cells supplemented with n-3 and n-6 polyunsaturated fatty acids. J Natl Cancer Inst 1986;77:1053-62.

[2]   Deschner EE, Lytle JS, Wong G, Ruperto JF, Newmark HL. The effect of dietary omega-3 fatty acids (fish oil) on azoxymethanol-induced focal areas of dysplasia and colon tumor incidence. Cancer 1990;66:2350-6.

[3]   Fernandes G, Friedrichs W, Schultz J, Venkatraman J. Modulation of MCF-7 tumor cell growth in nude mice by omega-3 fatty acid diet. Breast Cancer Res and Treat 1989;14:179.

[4]   Reddy BS, Sugie S. Effect of different levels of omega-3 and omega-6 fatty acids on azoxymethane-induced colon carcinogenesis in F344 rats. Cancer Res 1988;48:6642-7.

[5]   Rose DP, Connolly JM. Effects of dietary omega-3 fatty acids on human breast cancer growth and metastasis in nude mice. J Natl Cancer Inst 1993;85:1743-7.

[6]   Bougnoux P, Germain E, Chajes V, Hubert B, Lhuillery C, Le Flock O, Body G, Calais G. Cytotoxic drugs efficacy correlates with adipose tissue docosahexaenoic acid level in locally advanced breast carcinoma. Br J Cancer 1999;79(11):1765-9.

[7]   Barber MD, Fearon KCH, Tisdale MJ, McMillan DC, Ross JA. Effect of a fish oil-enriched nutritional supplement on metabolic mediators in patients with pancreatic cancer cachexia. Nutr Cancer 2001;40(2):118-24.

[8]   Li D, Ng A, Mann NJ, Sinclair A. Contribution of meat fat to dietary arachidonic acid. Lipids 1998;33:437-40.

[9]   de Gomez INT, Brenner RR. Oxidative desaturation of alpha-linolenic, linoleic and stearic acids by human liver microsomes. Lipids 1975;10:315-7.

[10]   Hague TA, Christoffersen BO. Effect of dietary fats on arachidonic acid and eicosapentaenoic acid biosynthesis and conversion of C22 fatty acids in isolated liver cells. Biochem Biophys Acta 1984;796:205-17.

[11]   Rose DP, Connolly JM. Omega-3 fatty acids as cancer chemopreventive agents. Pharmacology & Therapeutics 1999;83:217-44.

[12]   Balkwill F, Manzano LA. Inflammation and cancer: back to Virchow. Lancet 2001;357:539-45.

[13]   Williams CS, Mann M, Dubois RN. The role of cyclooxygenases in inflammation, cancer, and development. Oncogene 1999;18:7908-16.

[14]   Thun MJ, Henley SJ, Patrono C. Nonsteroidal anti-inflammatory drugs as anticancer agents: mechanistic, pharmacologic, and clinical issues. J Natl Cancer Inst 2002;94:252-66.

[15]   Hamid R, Singh J, Reddy BS, Cohen LA. Inhibition by dietary menhaden oil of cyclooxygenase-1 and-2 in N-nitrosomethylurea-induced rat mammary tumors. International Journal of Oncology 1999;14(3):523-8.

[16]   Obata T, Nagakura T, Masaki T, Maekawa K, Yamashita K. Eicosapentaenoic acid inhibits prostaglandin D2 generation by inhibiting cyclo-oxygenase-2 in cultured human mast cells. Clin Exp Allergy 1999;29(8):1129-35.

[17]   Needleman P, Raz A, Minkes MS, Ferrendelli JA, Specher H. Triene prostaglandins: prostacyclin and thromboxane biosynthesis and unique biological properties. Proc Natl Acad Sci USA 1979;76:944-8.

[18]   von Schacky C, Kiefl R, Marcus AJ, Broekman MJ, Kaminski WE. Dietary n-3 fatty acids accelerate catabolism of leukotriene B4 in human granulocytes. Biochim Biophys Acta 2004;1166:20-4.

[19]   Culp BR, Titus BG, Lands WE. Inhibition of prostaglandin biosynthesis by eicosapentaenoic acid. Prostaglandins Med 1979;3:269-78.

[20]   Marshall LA, Johnston PV. Modulation of tissue prostaglandin synthesizing capacity by increased ratios of dietary alpha-linolenic acid to linoleic acid. Lipids 1982;17:905-13.

[21]   Corey EJ, Shih C, Cashman JR. Docosahexaenoic acid is a strong inhibitor of prostaglandin but not leukotriene biosynthesis. Proc Natl Acad Sci USA 1983;80:3581-4.

[22]   Tsunomori M, Fujimoto Y, Muta E, Nishida H, Sakuma S, Fujita T. 15-Hydroperoxyeicosapentaenoic acid inhibits arachidonic acid metabolism in rabbit platelets more potently than eicosapentaenoic acid. Biochim Biophys Acta 1996;1300:171-6.

[23]   Hardman WE, Moyer MP, Cameron IL. Dietary fish oil sensitizes A549 lung xenografts to doxorubicin chemotherapy. Cancer Lett 2000;151:145-51.

[24]   Kimura Y. Carp Oil or Oleic Acid, but Not Linoleic Acid or Linolenic Acid, Inhibits Tumor Growth and Metastasis in Lewis Lung Carcinoma-Bearing Mice. J Nutr 2002 Jul;132(7):2069-75.

[25]   Calder PC, Davis J, Yaqoob P, Pala H, Thies F, Newsholme EA. Dietary fish oil suppresses human colon tumor growth in athymic mice. Clin Science 1998;94:303-11.

[26]   Chen ZY, Istfan NW. Docohexaenoic acid is a potent inducer of apoptosis in HT-29 colon cancer cells. Prostaglandins Leukot Essent Fatty Acids 2000;63(5):301-8.

[27]   Hardman WE, Barnes CJ, Knight CW, Cameron IL. Effects of iron supplementation and ET-18-OCH3 on MDA-MB 231 breast carcinomas in nude mice consuming a fish oil diet. Br J Cancer 1997;76:347-54.

[28]   Hardman WE, Moyer MP, Cameron IL. Fish oil supplementation enhanced CPT-11 (Irinotecan) efficacy against MCF7 breast carcinoma xenografts and ameliorated intestinal side effects. Br J Cancer 1999;81:440-8.

[29]   Connolly JM, Gilhooly EM, Rose DP. Effects of reduced dietary linoleic acid intake, alone or combined with an algae source of docosahexaenoic acid on MDA-MB-231 breast cancer cell growth and apoptosis in nude mice. Nutr Canc 1999;35(1):44-9.

[30]   Connolly JM, Coleman M, Rose DP. Effects of dietary fatty acids on DU145 human prostate cancer cell growth in athymic nude mice. Nutr Cancer 1997;29(2):114-9.

[31]   Hardman WE. Omega-3 fatty acids to augment cancer therapy. J Nutr 2002;132:3508S-12S.

[32]   Hardman WE, Avula CPR, Fernandes G, Cameron IL. Three percent dietary fish oil concentrate increased efficacy of doxorubicin against MDA-MB 231 human breast cancer xenografts. Clin Cancer Res 2001;7:2041-9.

[33]   de Salis HM, Meckling-Gill KA. EPA and DHA alter nucleoside drug and doxorubicin toxicity in L1210 cells but not in normal murine S1 macrophages. Cellular Pharmacology 1995;2:69-74.

[34]   Germain E, Lavandier F, Chajès V, Schubnel V, Bonnet P, Lhuillery C, Bougnoux P. Dietary n-3 polyunsaturated fatty acids and oxidants increase rat mammary tumor sensitivity to epirubicin without change in cardiac toxicity. Lipids 1999;34:S203.

[35]   Hochwald SN, Li J, Copeland EM, III, Moldawer LL, Lind DS, Mackay SL. Inhibition of NF-kB activiation potentiates the cytotoxicity of 5-FU and CPT-11 chemotherapy in human gastric cancer cells. Proc Am Assn Cancer Res 2002;43.

[36]   Shao Y, Pardini L, Pardini RS. Dietary menhaden oil enhances mitomycin C antitumor activity toward human mammary carcinoma MX-1. Lipids 1995;30:1035-45.

[37]   Cha MC, Meckling KA, Stewart C. Dietary docosahexaenoic acid levels influence the outcome of arabinosylcytosine chemotherapy in L1210 leukemic mice. Nutr Cancer 2002;44(2):176-81.

[38]   DeGraffenried LA, Friedrichs WE, Fulcher L, Fernandes G, Silva JM, Peralba JM, Hidalgo M. Eicosapentaenoic acid restores tamoxifen sensitivity in breast cancer cells with high Akt activity. Ann Oncology 2003;14(7):969-70.

[39]   Colas S, Paon L, Denis F, Prat M, Louisot P, Hoinard C, Le Floch O, Ogilvie G, Bougnoux P. Enhanced radiosensitivity of rat autochthonous mammary mamary tumor by dietary docosahexaenoic acid. Int J Cancer 2004;109(3):449-54.

[40]   Hardman WE, Moyer MP, Cameron IL. Small amounts of a concentrated omega-3 fatty acid product, INCELL AAFA, in the diet reduces the side-effects of the cancer chemotherapy drug, CPT-11 (irinotecan). Br J Cancer 2002;86:983-8.

[41]   Moses AW, Slater C, Preston T, Barber MD, Fearon KC. Reduced total energy expenditure and physical activity in cachexia patients with pancreatic cancer can be modulated by an energy and protein dense oral supplement enriched with n-3 fatty acids. Br J Cancer 2004;90(5):996-1002.

[42]   Vamvakas L, Kakolyris S, Kouroussis C, Kandilis K, Mavroudis D, Ziras N, Androulakis N, Kalbakis K, Sarra E, Souglakos J, Georgoulias V. Irinotecan (CPT-11) in combination with infusional 5-fluoracil and leucovorin (de Gramont regimen) as first-line treatment in patients with advanced colorectal cancer: a multicenter phase II study. Am J Clin Oncol 2002;25(1):65-70.

[43]   Sakai H, Sato T, Hamada N, Yasue M, Ikari A, Kakinoki B, Takeguchi N. Thromboxane A2, released by the anti-tumour drug irinotecan, is a novel stimulator of Cl-secretion in isolated rat colon. J Physiol 1997;505.1:133-44.

[44]   Sakai H, Diener M, Gartmann V, Takeguchi N. Eicosanoid-mediated Cl-secretion induced by the antitumor drug, irinotecan (CPT-11), in the rat colon. Naunyn-Schmiedeberg's Arch Pharmacol 1995;351:309-14.

[45]   Kase Y, Hayakawa T, Togashi Y, Kamataki T. Relevance of irinotecan hydrochloride diarrhea to the level of prostaglandin E2 and water absorbtion of large intestine in rats. Jpn J Pharmacol 1997;75:399-405.

[46]   Van Huyen J-PD, Bloch F, Attar A, Levoir D, Kreft C, Molina T, Brunk U. Diffuse mucosal damage in the large intestine associated with irinotecan (CPT-11). Dig Dis Sci 1998;43:2649-51.

[47]   Rothenberg ML, Cox JV, DeVore RF, Hainsworth JD, Pazdur R, Rivkin SE, Macdonald JS, Geyer CEJr, Sandbach J, Wolf DL, Mohrland JS, Elfring GL, Miller LL, Von Hoff DD. A multicenter, phase II trial of weekly irinotecan (CPT-11) in patients with previously treated colorectal carcinoma. Cancer 1999;85:786-95.

[48]   Rose DP, Connolly JM. Regulation of tumor angiogenesis by dietary fatty acids and eicosanoids. Nutr Cancer 2000;37(2):119-27.

[49]   Yang P, Felix E, Madden T, Chan D, Newman RA. Relative formation of PGE2 and PGE3 by eicosapentaenoic acid (EPA) and docosahexaenoic acid (DHA) in human lung cancer cells. Proc Am Assn Cancer Res 2002;43:number 1533.

[50]   Soslow RA, Dannenberg AJ, Rush D, Woerner BM, Khan KN, Masferrer J, Koki AT. COX-2 is expressed in human pulmonary, colonic and mammary tumors. Cancer 2000;89(12):2637-45.

[51]   Lanza-Jacoby S, Miller S, Flynn J, Gallatig K, Daskalakis C, Masferrer JL, Zweifel BS, Sembhi H, Russo IH. The cyclooxygenase-2 inhibitor, celecoxib, prevents the development of mammary tumors in Her-2/neu mice. Cancer Epidemiol Biomarkers & Prev 2003;12(12):1486-91.

[52]   Masferrer JL. Cyclooxygenase-2 inhibitors in cancer preventon and treatment. Adv Exp Med Biol 2003;532:209-13.

[53]   Blobe GC, Obeid LM, Hannun YA. Regulation of protein kinase C and role in cancer biology. Cancer Metastasis Rev 1994;13:411-431o.

[54]   Collett ED, Davidson LA, Fan Y-Y, Lupton JR, Chapkin RS. n-6 and n-3 polyunsaturated fatty acids differentially modulate oncogenic Ras activation in colonocytes. Am J Physiol Cell Physiol 2001;280:C1066-C1075.

[55]   Liu G, Bibus DM, Bode AM, Ma W-Y, Holman RT, Dong Z. Omega 3 but not omega 6 fatty acids inhibit AP-1 activity and cell transformation in JB6 cells. Proc Natl Acad Sci USA 2001;98(13):7510-5.

[56]   Abou-El-Ela SH, Prasse KW, Farrell RL, Carroll RW, Wade AE, Bunce OR. Effects of D,L-2-difluoromethylornithine and indomethicine on mammary tumor promotion in rats fed high n-3 and/or n-6 fat diets. Cancer Res 1989;49:1434-40.

[57]   Rose DP, Connolly JM. Effects of fatty acids and inhibitors of eicosanoid synthesis on the growth of a human breast cancer cell line in culture. Cancer Res 1990;50:7139-44.

[58]   Schwartz SA, Hernandez A, Evers BM. The role of NF-kB/IkB proteins in cancer; implications for novel treatment strategies. Surg Oncol 1999;8:143-53.

[59]   Connolly JM, Rose DP. Enhanced angiogenesis and growth of 12-lipoxygenase gene-transfected MCF-7 human breast cancer cells in athymic nude mice. Cancer Lett 1998;132:107-12.

[60]   Tsujii M, Dubois RN. Alterations in cellular adhesion and apoptosis in epithelial cells overexpression prostaglandin endoperoxide synthase 2. Cell 1995;83:493-501.

[61]   Chiu LCM, Wan JMF. Induction of apoptosis in HL-60 cells by eicosapentaenoic acid (EPA) is associated with downregulation of bcl-2 expression. Cancer Lett 1999;145:17-27.

[62]   Narayanan BA, Narayanan NK, Reddy BS. Docosahexaenoic acid regulated genes and transcription factors inducing apoptosis in human colon cancer cells. International Journal of Oncology 2001;19:1255-62.

[63]   Wang M, Liu YE, Ni J, Aygun B, Goldberg ID, Shi YE. Induction of mammary differentiation by mammary-derived Growth Inhibitor-related gene that interacts with an w-3 fatty acid on growth inhibition of breast cancer cells. Cancer Res 2000;60:6482-7.

[64]   Jones A, Harris AL. New developments in Angiogenesis: A major mechanism for Tumor Growth and Target for Therapy. Cancer J 1998;4(4):209-17.

[65]   Form DM, Auerbach R. PGE2 and angiogenesis. Proc Soc Exp Biol Med 1983;172:214-8.

[66]   McCarty MF. Fish oil may impede tumour angiogenesis and invasiveness by down-regulating protein kinase C and modulating eicosanoid production. Med Hypotheses 1996;46(2):107-15.

[67]   Tsujii M, Kawano S, Tsujii S, Sawaoka H, Hori M, Dubois RN. Cycloxygenase regulates angiogenesis induced by colon cancer cells. Cell 1998;93:705-16.

[68]   Tevar R, Jho DH, Babcock T, Helton WS, Espat NJ. Omega-3 fatty acid supplementation reduces tumor growth and vascular endothelial growth factor expression in a model of progressive non-metastasizing malignancy. J Parenter Enteral Nutr 2002;26(5):285-9.

[69]   Tsuji M, Murota SI, Morita I. Docosapentaenoic acid (22:5, n-3) suppresses tube-forming activity in endothelial cells induced by vascular endothelial growth factor. Prostaglandins Leukot Essent Fatty Acids 2003;68(5):337-42.

[70]   Kumar P, Miller AI, Polverini PJ. p38 MAPK mediates g-irradiation-induced endothelial cell apoptosis and VEGF protects endothelial cells through PI3K-Akt-Bcl-2 pathway. J Biol Chem 2004;papers in press (epub Aug 2).

[71]   Noble LS, Takayama K, Zeitoun KM, Putman JM, Johns DA, Hinshelwood MM, Agarwal VR, Zhao Y, Carr BR, Bulun SE. Prostaglandin E2 stimulates aromatase expression in endometriosis-derived stromal cells. J Clin Endoclrin Metab 1997;82:600-2.

[72]   Rao CV, Reddy BS. Modulating effect of amount and types of dietary fat on ornithine decarboxylase, tyrosine protein kinase and prostaglandin production during colon carconogenesis in male F344 rats. Carcinogenesis 1993;14:1327-33.

[73]   Bartram H, Gostner A, Scheppach W, Reddy BS, Rao CV, Dusel G, Richter F, Richter A, Kasper H. Effects of fish oil on rectal cell proliferation, mucosal fatty acids, and prostaglandin E2, release in healthy subjects. Gastroenterology 1993;105:1317-22.

[74]   Jump DB. Fatty acid regulation of gene transcription. Crit Rev Clin Lab Sci 2004;41(1):41-78.

[75]   Chen J, Stavro PM, Thompson LU. Dietary flaxseed inhibits human breast cancer growth and metastasis and downregulates expression of insulin-like growth factor and epidermal growth factor receptor. Nutr Canc 2002;43(2):187-92.

[76]   Connolly JM, Liu X-H, Rose DP. Dietary Linoleic acid-stimulated human breast cancer cell growth and metastasis in nude mice and their suppression by indomethacin, a cyclooxygenase inhibitor. Nutr Cancer 1996;25(3):231-40.

[77]   Karmali RA, Adams L, Trout JR. Plant and marine n-3 fatty acids inhibit experimental metastasis of rat mammary adenocarcinoma cells. Prostaglandins Leukot Essent Fatty Acids 1993;48:309-14.

[78]   Calle EE, Kaaks R. Overweight, obesity and cancer: epidemiological evidence and proposed mechanisms. Nature Reviews Cancer 2004;4(8):579-91.

[79]   Gelman L, Fruchart J-C, Auwerx J. An update on the mechanisms of action of the peroxisome proliferator-activated receptors (PPARs) and their roles in inflammation and cancer. Cell Mol Life Sci 1999;55:932-43.

[80]   Burns CP, Halabi S, Clamon GH, Hars V, Wagner BA, Hohl RJ, Lester E, Kirshner JJ, Vinciguerra V, Paskett E. Phase I clinical study of fish oil fatty acid capsules for patients with cancer cachexia: cancer and leukemia group B Study 9473. Clin Cancer Res 1999;5:3842-947.

[81]   Wigmore SJ, Ross JA, Falconer JS, Plester CE, Tisdale MJ, Carter DC, Fearon KCH. The effect of polyunsaturated fatty acids on the progress of cachexia in patients with pancreatic cancer. Nutrition 1996;12(Supp):S27-S30.

[82]   Jatoi A, Rowland K, Loprinzi CL, Sloan JA, Dakhil SR, MacDonald N, Gagnon B, Novotny PJ, Mailliard JA, Bushey TI, Nair S, Christensen B, North Central Cancer Treatment Group. An eicosapentaenoic acid supplement verses megestrol verses both for patients with cancer-assiciated wasting: a North Central Cancer Treatment Group and National Cancer Institute of Canada collaborative effort. J Clin Oncol 2004;22(12):2469-76.

[83]   Bougnoux P, Chajès V, Germain E, Hubert B, Lhuillery C, Le Floch O, Body G, Calais G. Cytotoxic drug efficacy correlates with adipose tissue docohexaenoic acid level in locally advanced breast carcinoma. Lipids 1999;34:S109.

[84]   Bagga D, Capone S, Wang H-J, Heber D, Lill M, Chap L, Glaspy JA. Dietary modulation of omega-3/omega-6 polyunsaturated fatty acid ratios in patients with breast cancer. J Natl Cancer Inst 1997;89(15):1123-31.

[85]   Simopoulos AP. The importance of the ratio of omega-6/omega-3 essential fatty acids. Biomed Pharmacother 2002 Oct;56(8):365-79.

[86]   Nelson GJ, Schmidt PS, Bartolini GL, Kelley DS, Kyle D. The effect of dietary docosahexaenoic acid on platelet function, platelet fatty acid composition and blood coagulation in humans. Lipids 1997;32(11):1129-36.

[87]   Simopoulos AP. Essential fatty acids in health and chronic disease. Am J Clin Nutr 1999;70:560S-9S.

CHAPTER 4

Green Tea Catechins and Cancer

Richard Egleton[*]

Nutrition and Cancer Center, Department of Pharmacology, Physiology and Toxicology, Joan C. Edward School of Medicine, Marshall University, Huntington, WV, USA

Abstract: Tea is one of the most widely consumed beverages in the world. Processed from the leaf of *Camellia* sinensis, teas contain a large number of phytochemicals including four catechins; epicatechin (EC), epigallocatechin (EGC), epicatechin gallate (ECG), and epigallocatechin gallate (EGCG). These catechins are at much higher levels in green tea compared to black tea. Over the last 20 years tea catechins have shown the potential for use as an adjunct therapy for a number of diseases including diabetes and cancer. This chapter will discuss the potential of green tea catechins in cancer prevention and as an adjunct to chemotherapy. Including the potential molecular mechanisms believed to be involved in regulating cancers.

Keywords: Caffeine, *Camellia Sinensis,* Cancer, Catechins, Diet, Epicatechin, Epicatechin Gallate, Epigallocatechin, Epigallocatechin Gallate, Food, Green Tea, Liver Cancer, Lung Cancer, Nutrition, Polyphenol, Prostate Cancer, Prostate Specific Antigen, Methylxanthines, Skin cancer, Tea, Theobromine, Theogallin, Theophylline.

INTRODUCTION

Tea is one of the most commonly consumed beverages world-wide. In the last 20 years a number of epidemiological studies have indicated that green tea in particular may have positive effects in both preventing or as an adjunct therapy in a number of diseases' including cardiovascular disease, metabolic syndrome and cancer [1-4]. Tea is produced from the leaf of *Camellia sinensis*, a bush grown in both tropical and subtropical regions of the world. There are 4 major types of tea consumed based on different manufacturing processes, black tea, green tea, oolong and white tea. To date most of the positive effects of tea have been linked to the consumption of green tea or green tea catechins, which will be the focus of this review. There are in the region of 4000 chemicals in green tea. The health-promoting effects of green tea have been linked largely to their high polyphenol content ~30-40% of the total dry weight (Table **1**.) Catechins are the predominant polyphenol and are comprised of epigallocatechin gallate (EGCG), epigallocatechin (EGC), epicatechin gallate (ECG), and epicatechin (EC) (Fig. **1**). EGCG is the most abundant of the catechins making up ~10% of the total dry weight of green tea [5]. A typical cup of green tea using 1g of leaf and 100 ml of water and brewed for 3 minutes will yield 250-300 mg of tea solids of which ~40 % are catechins [6].

The health benefits of green tea catechins are dependent on their oral bioavailability. Studies both in animals and humans have demonstrated that all four of the catechins are bioavailable orally from green tea and also when given individually (covered in detail in [7]). In general there is low uptake in the small intestine. This is in part due to the dimerization and degradation of the catechins at neutral pHs of the small intestine [8]. *In vitro* studies that mimicked the pH changes of the stomach and small intestine showed that all green tea catechins undergo degradation with the gallated catechins (EGCG, EGC and ECG) showing up to 80% loss compared to only a 10% loss for the non-gallated catechins [9]. This may be exacerbated by various foods [8]. In fact, human oral bioavailabilty studies show that fasting prior to administration can increase the peak plasma levels of EGCG ~5 fold [10].

*****Address Correspondence to Richard Egleton:** Nutrition and Cancer Center, Department of Pharmacology, Physiology and Toxicology, Joan C. Edwards School of Medicine, Marshall University, Byrd Biotechnology Science Center, Room 335H, 1700 Third Avenue, Huntington WV, 25755, USA; E-mail: egleton@marshall.edu

Pier Paolo Claudio and Richard M. Niles (Eds)

Table 1: Major components of green tea (adapted from [5])

Component	% Dry Weight
Polyphenols	30-42
Epigallocatechin gallate	11
Epicatechin gallate	2
Gallocatechin gallate	2
Epicatechin	10
Theogallin	2-3
Flavanols (quercetin/kaemferol/rutin)	5-10
Methylxanthines	7-9
Caffeine	3-5
Theophylline	0.02
Theobromine	0.01
Amino acids (theanine)	4-6
Organic Acids (quinic acid)	2

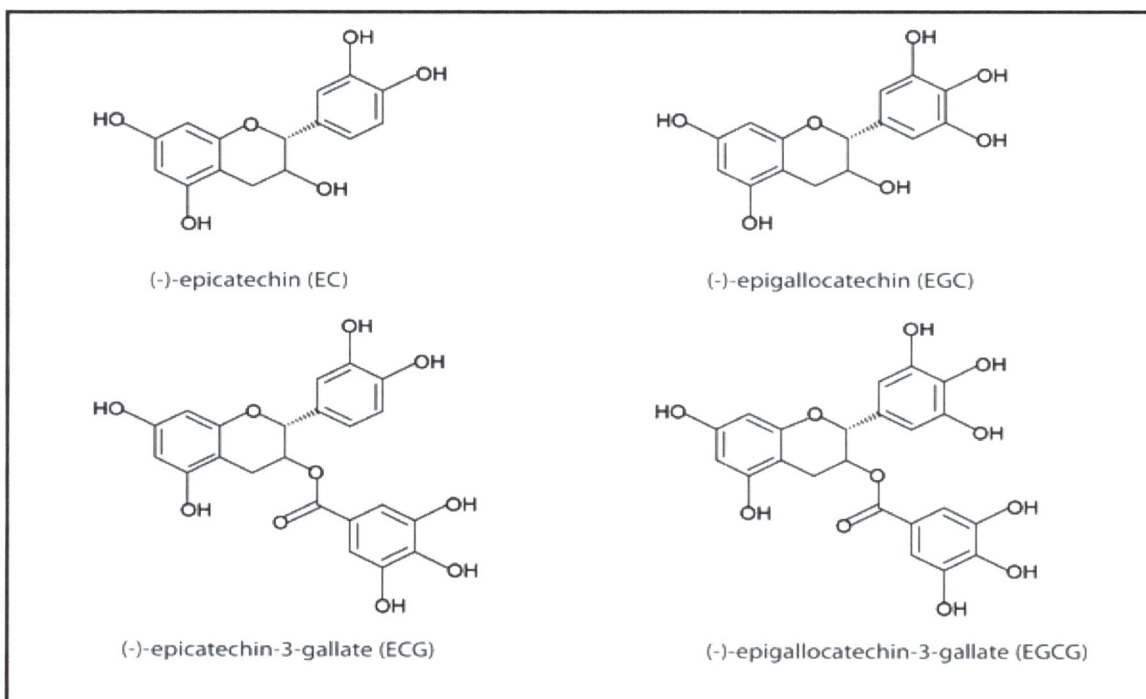

(-)-epicatechin (EC)

(-)-epigallocatechin (EGC)

(-)-epicatechin-3-gallate (ECG)

(-)-epigallocatechin-3-gallate (EGCG)

Figure 1: Structures of green tea catechins.

Interestingly as well as dimerization, there have also been reports of the formation of H_2O_2 at neutral pH [9], which could contribute to some of the effects of EGCG. In both animal and human studies, dietary green tea catechins have been shown to accumulate in tissues. A study looking at prostate accumulation of green tea catechins in C57BL/6 mice fed a green tea extract in their chow for two weeks showed an accumulation of all the major catechins ranging from ~0.1-5 nmol/g prostate tissue [11]. These levels rapidly declined on removal of the extract from the diet [11]. In a parallel human study in which participants drank green tea, there was also a significant accumulation of catechins in the prostate following a five day trial with levels ranging from 21-107 pmol/g prostate tissue [11]. Of particular interest from this study is that serum isolated from these patients following green tea therapy was able to slow down proliferation of the LNCaP prostate cancer cell line. In contrast pre green tea serum from the same patients did not [11]. These studies coupled with others indicate that green tea catechins are indeed bioavailable and can reach reasonable serum and tissue concentrations if given as a regular dietary supplement. Further studies have shown that EGCG at concentrations from 10-40 μmol/L dose dependently inhibits LNCaP cell proliferation [8]. In a single dose studies similar EGCG levels were recorded in human plasma following 1,200 mg of EGCG [10].

There is also a relatively rapid clearance of catechins from the system as evidenced by the above study in mice. Removals of the extract from the diet lead to a loss of the catechins from the system in under 24 hours [11]. Catechin metabolism and clearance is dependent on intestinal, microbial and hepatic metabolism. In the small intestine as mentioned above EGCG and EGC can undergo dimerization [9]. The catechins that do cross can be bioconjugated in both the intestinal Mucosa and the liver. This includes methylation, sulfation and glucoronidation. There appears to be a species difference in the bioconjugation process, for example EC in human liver/small intestine microsomes is largely sulfated with minimal if any glucoronidation. In contrast glucoronidation was the major form of bioconjugation in rat liver microsomes [12]. Those catechins that are not taken up at the small intestine, can be metabolized by the gut flora in the large intestine into an array of aromatic acids, which can be further metabolized to benzoic acid derivatives [7]. These benzoic acid derivatives can then be absorbed and conjugated with glycine, glucoronidation and sulfation by the liver [8]. The metabolism profiles of the catechins is important as it not only effects the route of elimination (renal *vs.* billary), but several of the metabolites are active. For example the 5 and 7-O-methyl epicatechins do not protect fibroblasts or neurons from oxidative stress. In contrast epicatechin and methylepicatechin do [13]. It is also important to note that due to the rapid clearance it is unlikely that metabolites will build up in the system, unless there is a prolonged and frequent administration of green tea catechins [14]. Thus any use of either green tea or EGCG should be as a prolonged treatment rather than single or short term administration.

MECHANISM OF ACTION

There are several mechanisms of action for the polyphenolic compounds from green tea, which make them an attractive potential adjunct in cancer therapy. These include H_2O_2 production, anti-oxidant capacity, anti-angiogenic, anti-mutagenic, anti-inflammatory, induction of apoptosis and cell cycle arrest [15]. To date most studies have concentrated on the mechanism of EGCG and that will be the focus of this section. It has become apparent that EGCG can interfere with multiple signaling cascades. This includes receptor tyrosine kinase (RTK) signaling leading to numerous effects including reducing NFκB and Ap-1 induced transcription. EGCG can also bind directly to the HSP 90 of the cytoplasmic Aryl hydrocarbon receptor (AhR) complex, resulting in reduced AhR transcription, and also potentially reduced AhR mediated ubiquitination. Finally EGCG can bind to the lamanin 67kDa receptor, and thus regulate the cytoskeleton.

Several studies have shown that EGCG regulates the activity of RTKs including members of the erbB family of receptors. The erbB family includes epidermal growth factor receptor (EGFR) as well as the HER2 and HER3 receptors and thus blocking of these receptors has obvious utility in cancer. EGCG blocks EGF binding to the EGFR thus preventing activation of the tyrosine kinase [16]. Subsequent studies have shown that EGCG also inhibits the activation of HER2 and HER3 [17, 18], in various human cancer cell lines. Inhibition of these receptors leads to a decrease in ERK activity, reduction in Cyclin D-1 and Bcl-xl levels, thus making the cells more prone to apoptosis [15]. Inhibition of growth factor mediated activation of AP-1 and NF-κB mediated transcription *via* EGCG has also been reported [19].

Other growth factors that are regulated *via* EGCG include the IGF and VEGF systems. IGF and its receptors is an important factor in the growth of various cancers. EGCG treatment leads to an increased ratio of IGF binding protein-3 (IGFBP-3) to the levels of both IGF-1 and 2, with a net effect of reduced IGF signaling [20, 21]. VEGFs receptor signaling is also modulated by EGCG. EGCG inhibits VGEF induced autophosphorylation of its primary receptors Flk-1 and Flt-1 [22] and prevents VEGF receptor complex formation [23]. This results in a reduction of VEGF induced DNA synthesis and reduced cell proliferation [24]. VEGF is a key regulator of angiogenesis in tumors [25]. Regulation of these RTK's can obviously have a significant effect of activation of signaling cascades. It has however become apparent that

EGCG can directly regulate a number of these cascades, thus magnifying the response. Several studies have shown that EGCG can inhibit the activity of ERK, AKT, Phospho-ERK and MAPK [26-31]. Inhibition of these kinases will significantly affect cellular signaling and transcription (Fig. **2**.). EGCGs inhibition of kinase cascades can lead to a reduction in JNK, AP-1, NFκβ [28, 32-35] and subsequent transcription of genes essential for cancer growth and metastasis including matrix metaloproteases [34, 35], cyclin D1 [17, 36], Cox-2 [18, 37] and multidrug efflux transporters [38].

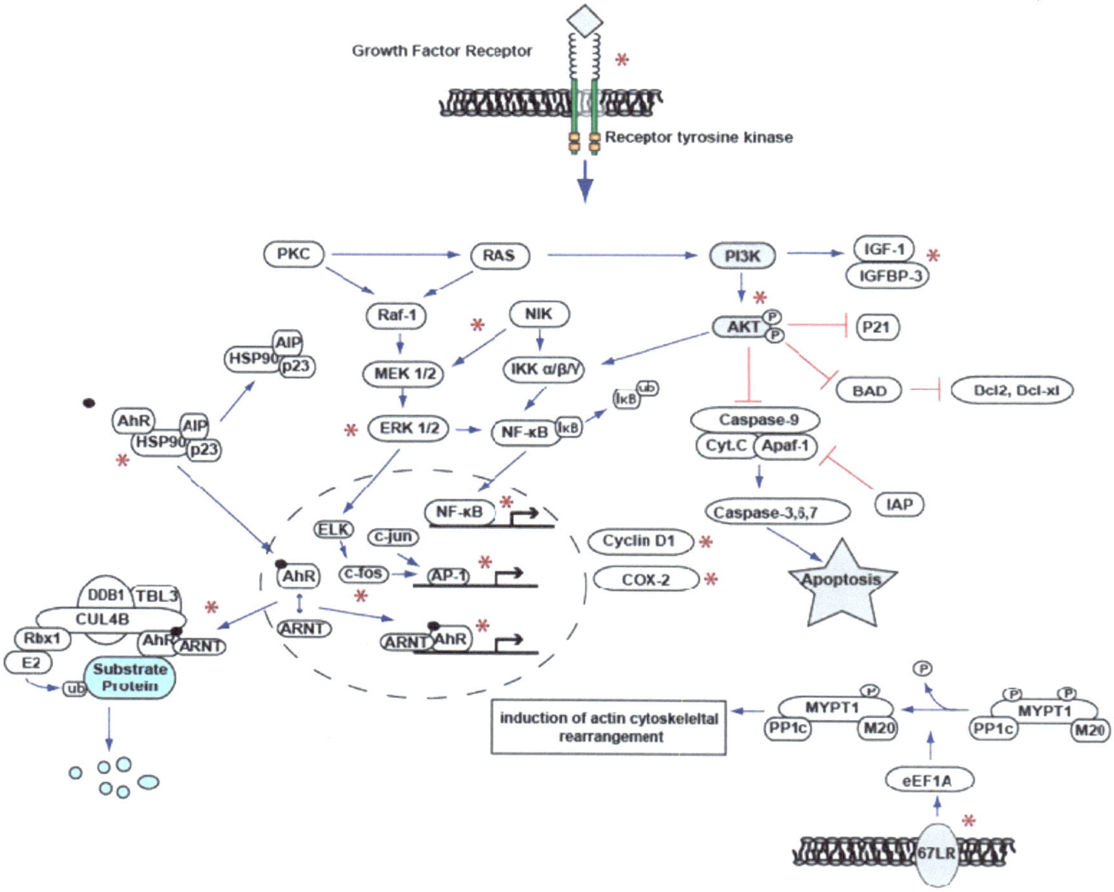

Figure 2: Signaling pathways that are modulated by EGCG. Sites at which EGCG is known to interact are indicated with a *. Figure is based on the papers outlined in the text.

More recent studies have shown two other mechanisms of EGCG activity. EGCG has been shown to act as an inhibitor of the arylhydrocarbon receptor (AhR) *via* its interaction with heat shock protein 90 [39, 40]. EGCG does not prevent AhR ligand binding, but it does prevent the dissociation of AhR from HSP90 following binding [40]. Once AhR has been released by HSP90, it will either interact with the AhR nuclear translocator (ARNT) [41], or will become part of an E3 ubiquitin ligase complex [42] (see Fig. **2**). Inhibiting either of these actions can have a significant effect in cancer treatment. The AhR transcription factor complex plays an important role in regulating the expression of phase I and phase II metabolism enzymes and also in the regulation of multidrug resistance. Inhibition of this complex will reduce the expression of various cytochrome P450 enzymes as well as P-glycoprotein and MRP-2 [43, 44], reduce matrix remodeling [45] and regulate estrogen receptor signaling [42, 45]. This combination of effects should reduce metastatic properties of tumors and also increase their sensitivity to chemotherapy.

Other studies have recently shown that EGCG is a substrate for the 67kDa laminin receptor [46-48]. EGCG binding to the 67LR is believed to lead to the activation of myosin phosphatase, this in turn leads to an actin cytoskeleton rearrangement that leads to cell growth inhibition [47].

USES IN CANCER THERAPY

Based on the interactions described in the above section, it is apparent that ECGC could play a significant role in prevention of cancer and also in cancer therapy. In fact over the last 20 years, green tea catechins have been proposed as an adjunct therapy in numerous cancers including skin, liver, lung, breast, prostate and various hematological disorders. The following sections will skim over some of the studies that have reported clinical, epidemiological, animal and cell effects of EGCG.

Skin Cancer

Studies have shown that EGCG could inhibit UVB-induced erythema, oxidative stress in human skin [49]. Further, EGCG also prevented UVB-induction of mediators believed to be responsible for skin cancer induction [49]. In cell studies, normal human epidermal keratinocytes were protected from UVB induced DNA damage by EGCG [50]. EGCG also inhibited proliferation and colony forming of melanoma cell lines (A-375 & Hs-294T) [36]. In animal models purified green tea polyphenol mixtures prevented UVB and photocarcinogenesis in mice [51, 52]. Green tea polyphenols also reduced both tumor load and onset in the DMBA treated mouse skin tumors [53]. There have also been several studies that have implicated that EGCG can either slow progression or sensitize tumors to therapy. Green tea polyphenols reduced malignant conversion of papillomas to squamous cell carcinomas in a mouse model [54]. EGCG also sensitized melanoma tumors to IFN, leading to reduced tumor size and PCNA production in nude athymic mice [55].

Liver Cancer

Several studies have shown that the incidence of liver cancer is reduced in green tea drinkers in both Japan and China [56, 57], indicating that some constituent of green tea is protective. In animal models oral EGCG has been shown to induce apoptosis in human hepatocellular carcinoma (HCC) cell line HLE xenograft model in mice [58]. Subsequent *in vitro* studies indicate that this was due to a decrease in Bcl-2α and Bcl-xl levels probably due to an inactivation of NF-κβ [58]. Similar results were seen with a number of other human liver cancer cell lines including HEPG2, HuH-7 and PLC/PRF/5 cells [58]. Various other green tea catechins have also been shown to reduce HEPG2 cell numbers [59, 60]. In hepatocarcinoma SMMC7721 cells, EGCG leads to a rapid apoptosis in part due to an attenuation of mitochondrial transmembrane potentials, the alteration of Bcl-2 family proteins and increased ROS production [61]. Inhibition of VEGF signaling has also been indicated in the growth inhibition of HCC cells both *in vitro* and *in vivo* [62], and could also inhibit thrombin induced invasiveness [63]. EGCG can also sensitize carcinoma cells to doxorubicin *via* a reduction in the expression of P-gp [64].

Lung Cancer

Epidemiological studies indicate that Green tea consumption reduces the risk of lung cancer [65]. Though interestingly this does not seem to be the case for smokers [66]. In animal models EGCG has been reported to reduce tumor load in tobacco tumorogenesis models [67]. Green tea has also been reported to reduce metastasis of mouse lung carcinomas [68]. There is evidence that the complex mixtures found in Polyphenon E rather than pure EGCG are more effective at reducing tumor multiplicity [69, 70]. *In vitro* EGCG reduces the proliferation several non-small cell cancer cell lines [71]. In drug resistant lung cancer cells EGCG can induce apoptosis by inhibiting telomerase activity [72]. EGCG has also been reported to inhibit 95-D cell invasion in invasion assays *via* reduction of MMP-9 levels and preventing NF-κβ nuclear translocation [73].

Breast Cancer

Green tea consumption in general has been linked with a reduction in risk for breast cancer [74-76]. Further it has been linked to a reduction in the rate of reoccurrence of breast cancer [77]. Experimentally various green tea catechins have been show to induce cell death in breast cancer cell lines such as MCF-7 [59]. For EGCG, this is probably in part due to the reduced expression of both HSP-70 and 90 [78]. There is also a reduction of colony formation both in soft agar and in mouse xenograft studies with MCF-7 cells [78]. Reduction of MMP levels has also been reported due to a reduction in kinase activity that leads to a lowered transcriptional activity of NF-κβ [79].

Prostate Cancer

Epidemiology studies indicate that green tea is protective against prostate cancer in Chinese [80, 81], but not Japanese males [82]. Clinically green tea catechins have been shown to reduce conversion of high-grade prostatic intraepithelial neoplasia to prostatic cancer in patients for up to 24 months [83, 84]. Further EGCG has been shown to reduce the serum levels of VEGF, PSA and hepatocyte growth factor (HGF) in prostate cancer patients [85] as well as *in vitro* [85]. Interestingly, though as noted above in Japanese males green tea consumption did not protect against localized prostate cancer, there is a dose dependent decrease in the risk of advanced prostate cancer [86]. In the TRAMP mouse modes it is apparent that EGCG is more effective at inhibiting early stage prostate cancer than late stage [87, 88]. The probable mechanism of early stage inhibition is a reduction in both androgen and growth factor receptor expression and reduced intracellular kinase levels [88]. Other studies in the TRAMP model have also shown that green tea will induce prostate cancer cell apoptosis and significantly reduce metastases [89]. Cell studies indicate several potential mechanisms for the efficacy of EGCG in prostate cancer including inhibition of fatty acid synthase [90], downregulation of NF-κβ [91], decreased PI3Kinase activity and decreased phospho-AKT [91], suppression of androgen receptor signaling [92], and chromatin remodeling [93].

Hematological

Several studies indicate that green tea consumption can reduce the risk of leukemia [94, 95]. In fact the risk of hematological malignancies was inversely proportional to the levels of green tea consumed [96]. In a group of patients with low grade B-cell malignances, green tea supplements lead to a "partial response" as defined by standard response criteria [97]. This has lead to a phase I clinical trial with polyphenon E in which patients showed minimal adverse effects [98]. The study also reported several positive effects of EGCG including a 20% reduction in absolute lymphocyte count, and in those patients with palpable adenopathy, a reduction in the sum of nodal areas [98]. In cell culture studies the EGCG was shown to induce cell death of acute myeloid leukemia cells isolated from patients *via* a 67 kDa laminin receptor mediated mechanism [99, 100]. The EGCG was also shown to be only effective against cancer cells [100]. Subsequent studies with HL-60 cells indicate this may be due to the loss of the 67 kDa receptor during differentiation, which leads to a protection against EGCG [100]. The mechanism is in part due to a reduction of BCL-2 and an activation of Caspase-3 that induces apoptosis [101]. EGCG has been reported to sensitize cancers to various chemotherapeutic agents, however several studies have shown that it will actually inhibits the action of bortezomib [102, 103]. Bortezomib is a boron containing proteasome inhibitor used in multiple myeloma, other boron containing proteasome inhibitors also were inhibited by EGCG, while proteasome inhibitors without boron were not [102]. Other groups however have not seen the same response of EGCG and bortezomib [104].

CONCLUSIONS

Green tea, has been lauded as a "wonder herb". To a certain degree green tea has shown promise as a prophylactic and also in clinical studies in several types of cancer. The epidemiological studies have largely focused on Asian populations that have been ingesting green tea for decades, based on the metabolism of green tea catechins, it is likely that any long term prophylactic benefit would require use for several years. Also few studies have looked at how either menopause or pregnancy could affect EGCG action. One of EGCG's actions is *via* the AhR, a transcription factor heavily involved in regulation of estrogen receptors. Caution should also be taken when considering either green tea, or its major catechin EGCG in patients due to the large number of systems that it can interact with. EGCG can lead to the down regulation of several phase I and II metabolizing enzymes as well as the efflux transporters. Thus the potential for drug-drug interactions is very high. In the controlled clinical settings this is less worrying however, due to the ability of patients to access the web and a huge amount of data on EGCG, it is likely that they will self medicate with EGCG without informing clinicians. This could lead to some potentially toxic changes in pharmacokinetics. Further EGCG seems to reduce the efficacy of at least one type of drug (boron containing proteasome inhibitors), which could lead to reducing efficacy of treatment. Despite these caveats, the potential for EGCG or drugs developed from this catechin in cancer therapy is significant.

REFERENCES

[1]   Boehm K, Borrelli F, Ernst E, Habacher G, Hung SK, Milazzo S, *et al.* Green tea (Camellia sinensis) for the prevention of cancer. Cochrane Database Syst Rev 2009 (3): CD005004.

[2]   Thielecke F, Boschmann M. The potential role of green tea catechins in the prevention of the metabolic syndrome-a review. Phytochemistry 2009; 70(1): 11-24.

[3]   Wolfram S. Effects of green tea and EGCG on cardiovascular and metabolic health. J Am Coll Nutr. 2007; 26(4): 373S-88S.

[4]   Yang CS, Wang X, Lu G, Picinich SC. Cancer prevention by tea: animal studies, molecular mechanisms and human relevance. Nat Rev Cancer 2009; 9(6): 429-39.

[5]   Dufresne CJ, Farnworth ER. A review of latest research findings on the health promotion properties of tea. J Nutr Biochem 2001; 12(7): 404-21.

[6]   Mukhtar H, Ahmad N. Cancer chemoprevention: future holds in multiple agents. Toxicol Appl Pharmacol 1999; 158(3): 207-10.

[7]   de Mejia EG, Ramirez-Mares MV, Puangpraphant S. Bioactive components of tea: cancer, inflammation and behavior. Brain Behav Immun 2009; 23(6): 721-31.

[8]   Henning SM, Choo JJ, Heber D. Nongallated compared with gallated flavan-3-ols in green and black tea are more bioavailable. J Nutr 2008; 138(8): 1529S-34S.

[9]   Neilson AP, Hopf AS, Cooper BR, Pereira MA, Bomser JA, Ferruzzi MG. Catechin degradation with concurrent formation of homo-and heterocatechin dimers during *in vitro* digestion. J Agric Food Chem 2007; 55(22): 8941-9.

[10]   Chow HH, Hakim IA, Vining DR, Crowell JA, Ranger-Moore J, Chew WM, *et al.* Effects of dosing condition on the oral bioavailability of green tea catechins after single-dose administration of Polyphenon E in healthy individuals. Clin Cancer Res 2005; 11(12): 4627-33.

[11]   Henning SM, Aronson W, Niu Y, Conde F, Lee NH, Seeram NP, *et al.* Tea polyphenols and theaflavins are present in prostate tissue of humans and mice after green and black tea consumption. J Nutr 2006; 136(7): 1839-43.

[12]   Vaidyanathan JB, Walle T. Glucuronidation and sulfation of the tea flavonoid (-)-epicatechin by the human and rat enzymes. Drug Metab Dispos 2002; 30(8): 897-903.

[13]   Spencer JP, Schroeter H, Crossthwaithe AJ, Kuhnle G, Williams RJ, Rice-Evans C. Contrasting influences of glucuronidation and O-methylation of epicatechin on hydrogen peroxide-induced cell death in neurons and fibroblasts. Free Radic Biol Med 2001; 31(9): 1139-46.

[14]   Manach C, Scalbert A, Morand C, Remesy C, Jimenez L. Polyphenols: food sources and bioavailability. Am J Clin Nutr 2004; 79(5): 727-47.

[15]   Shimizu M, Shirakami Y, Moriwaki H. Targeting receptor tyrosine kinases for chemoprevention by green tea catechin, EGCG. Int J Mol Sci 2008; 9(6): 1034-49.

[16]   Liang YC, Lin-shiau SY, Chen CF, Lin JK. Suppression of extracellular signals and cell proliferation through EGF receptor binding by (-)-epigallocatechin gallate in human A431 epidermoid carcinoma cells. J Cell Biochem 1997; 67(1): 55-65.

[17]   Masuda M, Suzui M, Lim JT, Weinstein IB. Epigallocatechin-3-gallate inhibits activation of HER-2/neu and downstream signaling pathways in human head and neck and breast carcinoma cells. Clin Cancer Res 2003; 9(9): 3486-91.

[18]   Shimizu M, Deguchi A, Joe AK, McKoy JF, Moriwaki H, Weinstein IB. EGCG inhibits activation of HER3 and expression of cyclooxygenase-2 in human colon cancer cells. J Exp Ther Oncol 2005; 5(1): 69-78.

[19]   Shimizu M, Deguchi A, Lim JT, Moriwaki H, Kopelovich L, Weinstein IB. (-)-Epigallocatechin gallate and polyphenon E inhibit growth and activation of the epidermal growth factor receptor and human epidermal growth factor receptor-2 signaling pathways in human colon cancer cells. Clin Cancer Res 2005; 11(7): 2735-46.

[20]   Shimizu M, Deguchi A, Hara Y, Moriwaki H, Weinstein IB. EGCG inhibits activation of the insulin-like growth factor-1 receptor in human colon cancer cells. Biochem Biophys Res Commun 2005; 334(3): 947-53.

[21]   Shimizu M, Shirakami Y, Sakai H, Tatebe H, Nakagawa T, Hara Y, *et al.* EGCG inhibits activation of the insulin-like growth factor (IGF)/IGF-1 receptor axis in human hepatocellular carcinoma cells. Cancer Lett 2007 Dec 28.

[22]   Lee YK, Bone ND, Strege AK, Shanafelt TD, Jelinek DF, Kay NE. VEGF receptor phosphorylation status and apoptosis is modulated by a green tea component, epigallocatechin-3-gallate (EGCG), in B-cell chronic lymphocytic leukemia. Blood 2004; 104(3): 788-94.

[23]   Rodriguez SK, Guo W, Liu L, Band MA, Paulson EK, Meydani M. Green tea catechin, epigallocatechin-3-gallate, inhibits vascular endothelial growth factor angiogenic signaling by disrupting the formation of a receptor complex. Int J Cancer 2006; 118(7): 1635-44.

[24]   Neuhaus T, Pabst S, Stier S, Weber AA, Schror K, Sachinidis A, *et al.* Inhibition of the vascular-endothelial growth factor-induced intracellular signaling and mitogenesis of human endothelial cells by epigallocatechin-3 gallate. Eur J Pharmacol 2004; 483(2-3): 223-7.

[25]   Bussolati B, Deregibus MC, Camussi G. Characterization of molecular and functional alterations of tumor endothelial cells to design anti-angiogenic strategies. Curr Vasc Pharmacol 2010; 8(2):220-32.

[26]   Chung JY, Park JO, Phyu H, Dong Z, Yang CS. Mechanisms of inhibition of the Ras-MAP kinase signaling pathway in 30.7b Ras 12 cells by tea polyphenols (-)-epigallocatechin-3-gallate and theaflavin-3,3'-digallate. FASEB J 2001; 15(11): 2022-4.

[27]   Kundu JK, Na HK, Chun KS, Kim YK, Lee SJ, Lee SS, *et al.* Inhibition of phorbol ester-induced COX-2 expression by epigallocatechin gallate in mouse skin and cultured human mammary epithelial cells. J Nutr 2003; 133(11 Suppl 1): 3805S-10S.

[28]   Kundu JK, Surh YJ. Epigallocatechin gallate inhibits phorbol ester-induced activation of NF-kappa B and CREB in mouse skin: role of p38 MAPK. Ann N Y Acad Sci 2007; 1095: 504-12.

[29]   Sah JF, Balasubramanian S, Eckert RL, Rorke EA. Epigallocatechin-3-gallate inhibits epidermal growth factor receptor signaling pathway. Evidence for direct inhibition of ERK1/2 and AKT kinases. J Biol Chem 2004; 279(13): 12755-62.

[30]   Shankar S, Chen Q, Srivastava RK. Inhibition of PI3K/AKT and MEK/ERK pathways act synergistically to enhance antiangiogenic effects of EGCG through activation of FOXO transcription factor. J Mol Signal 2008; 3: 7.

[31]   Deguchi H, Fujii T, Nakagawa S, Koga T, Shirouzu K. Analysis of cell growth inhibitory effects of catechin through MAPK in human breast cancer cell line T47D. Int J Oncol 2002; 21(6): 1301-5.

[32]   Kim SJ, Jeong HJ, Lee KM, Myung NY, An NH, Yang WM, *et al.* Epigallocatechin-3-gallate suppresses NF-kappaB activation and phosphorylation of p38 MAPK and JNK in human astrocytoma U373MG cells. J Nutr Biochem 2007; 18(9): 587-96.

[33]   Singh R, Ahmed S, Malemud CJ, Goldberg VM, Haqqi TM. Epigallocatechin-3-gallate selectively inhibits interleukin-1beta-induced activation of mitogen activated protein kinase subgroup c-Jun N-terminal kinase in human osteoarthritis chondrocytes. J Orthop Res 2003; 21(1): 102-9.

[34]   Vayalil PK, Katiyar SK. Treatment of epigallocatechin-3-gallate inhibits matrix metalloproteinases-2 and-9 *via* inhibition of activation of mitogen-activated protein kinases, c-jun and NF-kappaB in human prostate carcinoma DU-145 cells. Prostate 2004; 59(1): 33-42.

[35]   Yun HJ, Yoo WH, Han MK, Lee YR, Kim JS, Lee SI. Epigallocatechin-3-gallate suppresses TNF-alpha-induced production of MMP-1 and-3 in rheumatoid arthritis synovial fibroblasts. Rheumatol Int 2008; 29(1): 23-9.

[36]   Nihal M, Ahmad N, Mukhtar H, Wood GS. Anti-proliferative and proapoptotic effects of (-)-epigallocatechin-3-gallate on human melanoma: possible implications for the chemoprevention of melanoma. Int J Cancer 2005; 114(4): 513-21.

[37]   Peng G, Dixon DA, Muga SJ, Smith TJ, Wargovich MJ. Green tea polyphenol (-)-epigallocatechin-3-gallate inhibits cyclooxygenase-2 expression in colon carcinogenesis. Mol Carcinog 2006; 45(5): 309-19.

[38]   Farabegoli F, Papi A, Bartolini G, Ostan R, Orlandi M. (-)-Epigallocatechin-3-gallate downregulates Pg-P and BCRP in a tamoxifen resistant MCF-7 cell line. Phytomedicine 2010; 17(5): 356-62.

[39]   Palermo CM, Westlake CA, Gasiewicz TA. Epigallocatechin gallate inhibits aryl hydrocarbon receptor gene transcription through an indirect mechanism involving binding to a 90 kDa heat shock protein. Biochemistry 2005; 44(13): 5041-52.

[40]   Yin Z, Henry EC, Gasiewicz TA. (-)-Epigallocatechin-3-gallate is a novel Hsp90 inhibitor. Biochemistry. 2009 Jan 20;48(2):336-45.

[41]   Swedenborg E, Pongratz I. AhR and ARNT modulate ER signaling. Toxicology 2010; 268(3): 132-8.

[42]   Ohtake F, Fujii-Kuriyama Y, Kato S. AhR acts as an E3 ubiquitin ligase to modulate steroid receptor functions. Biochem Pharmacol 2009; 77(4): 474-84.

[43]   Swanson HI. Cytochrome P450 expression in human keratinocytes: an aryl hydrocarbon receptor perspective. Chem Biol Interact 2004; 149(2-3): 69-79.

[44]   Klaassen CD, Slitt AL. Regulation of hepatic transporters by xenobiotic receptors. Curr Drug Metab 2005; 6(4): 309-28.

[45]   Kung T, Murphy KA, White LA. The aryl hydrocarbon receptor (AhR) pathway as a regulatory pathway for cell adhesion and matrix metabolism. Biochem Pharmacol 2009; 77(4): 536-46.

[46]   Umeda D, Tachibana H, Yamada K. Epigallocatechin-3-O-gallate disrupts stress fibers and the contractile ring by reducing myosin regulatory light chain phosphorylation mediated through the target molecule 67 kDa laminin receptor. Biochem Biophys Res Commun 2005; 333(2): 628-35.

[47]   Umeda D, Yano S, Yamada K, Tachibana H. Green tea polyphenol epigallocatechin-3-gallate signaling pathway through 67-kDa laminin receptor. J Biol Chem 2008; 283(6): 3050-8.

[48]   Wang CT, Chang HH, Hsiao CH, Lee MJ, Ku HC, Hu YJ, *et al.* The effects of green tea (-)-epigallocatechin-3-gallate on reactive oxygen species in 3T3-L1 preadipocytes and adipocytes depend on the glutathione and 67 kDa laminin receptor pathways. Mol Nutr Food Res 2009;53(3): 349-60.

[49]   Katiyar SK. Skin photoprotection by green tea: antioxidant and immunomodulatory effects. Curr Drug Targets Immune Endocr Metabol Disord 2003; 3(3): 234-42.

[50]   Morley N, Clifford T, Salter L, Campbell S, Gould D, Curnow A. The green tea polyphenol (-)-epigallocatechin gallate and green tea can protect human cellular DNA from ultraviolet and visible radiation-induced damage. Photodermatol Photoimmunol Photomed 2005; 21(1): 15-22.

[51]   Meeran SM, Akhtar S, Katiyar SK. Inhibition of UVB-induced skin tumor development by drinking green tea polyphenols is mediated through DNA repair and subsequent inhibition of inflammation. J Invest Dermatol 2009; 129(5): 1258-70.

[52]   Gensler HL, Timmermann BN, Valcic S, Wachter GA, Dorr R, Dvorakova K, *et al.* Prevention of photocarcinogenesis by topical administration of pure epigallocatechin gallate isolated from green tea. Nutr Cancer 1996; 26(3): 325-35.

[53]   Roy P, Nigam N, George J, Srivastava S, Shukla Y. Induction of apoptosis by tea polyphenols mediated through mitochondrial cell death pathway in mouse skin tumors. Cancer Biol Ther 2009; 8(13): 1281-7.

[54]   Katiyar SK, Mohan RR, Agarwal R, Mukhtar H. Protection against induction of mouse skin papillomas with low and high risk of conversion to malignancy by green tea polyphenols. Carcinogenesis 1997; 18(3): 497-502.

[55]   Nihal M, Ahsan H, Siddiqui IA, Mukhtar H, Ahmad N, Wood GS. (-)-Epigallocatechin-3-gallate (EGCG) sensitizes melanoma cells to interferon induced growth inhibition in a mouse model of human melanoma. Cell Cycle 2009; 8(13): 2057-63.

[56]   Jin X, Zheng RH, Li YM. Green tea consumption and liver disease: a systematic review. Liver Int 2008; 28(7): 990-6.

[57]   Ui A, Kuriyama S, Kakizaki M, Sone T, Nakaya N, Ohmori-Matsuda K, *et al.* Green tea consumption and the risk of liver cancer in Japan: the Ohsaki Cohort study. Cancer Causes Control 2009; 20(10): 1939-45.

[58]   Nishikawa T, Nakajima T, Moriguchi M, Jo M, Sekoguchi S, Ishii M, *et al.* A green tea polyphenol, epigalocatechin-3-gallate, induces apoptosis of human hepatocellular carcinoma, possibly through inhibition of Bcl-2 family proteins. J Hepatol 2006; 44(6): 1074-82.

[59]   Friedman M, Mackey BE, Kim HJ, Lee IS, Lee KR, Lee SU, *et al.* Structure-activity relationships of tea compounds against human cancer cells. J Agric Food Chem 2007; 55(2): 243-53.

[60]   Uesato S, Kitagawa Y, Kamishimoto M, Kumagai A, Hori H, Nagasawa H. Inhibition of green tea catechins against the growth of cancerous human colon and hepatic epithelial cells. Cancer Lett 2001; 170(1): 41-4.

[61]   Li W, Nie S, Yu Q, Xie M. (-)-Epigallocatechin-3-gallate induces apoptosis of human hepatoma cells by mitochondrial pathways related to reactive oxygen species. J Agric Food Chem 2009; 57(15): 6685-91.

[62]   Shirakami Y, Shimizu M, Adachi S, Sakai H, Nakagawa T, Yasuda Y, *et al.* (-)-Epigallocatechin gallate suppresses the growth of human hepatocellular carcinoma cells by inhibiting activation of the vascular endothelial growth factor-vascular endothelial growth factor receptor axis. Cancer Sci 2009; 100(10): 1957-62.

[63]   Kaufmann R, Henklein P, Settmacher U. Green tea polyphenol epigallocatechin-3-gallate inhibits thrombin-induced hepatocellular carcinoma cell invasion and p42/p44-MAPKinase activation. Oncol Rep 2009; 21(5): 1261-7.

[64]   Liang G, Tang A, Lin X, Li L, Zhang S, Huang Z, *et al.* Green tea catechins augment the antitumor activity of doxorubicin in an *in vivo* mouse model for chemoresistant liver cancer. Int J Oncol 2010; 37(1): 111-23.

[65]   Tang N, Wu Y, Zhou B, Wang B, Yu R. Green tea, black tea consumption and risk of lung cancer: a meta-analysis. Lung Cancer 2009; 65(3): 274-83.

[66]   Zhong L, Goldberg MS, Gao YT, Hanley JA, Parent ME, Jin F. A population-based case-control study of lung cancer and green tea consumption among women living in Shanghai, China. Epidemiology 2001 Nov; 12(6): 695-700.

[67]   Xu Y, Ho CT, Amin SG, Han C, Chung FL. Inhibition of tobacco-specific nitrosamine-induced lung tumorigenesis in A/J mice by green tea and its major polyphenol as antioxidants. Cancer Res 1992; 52(14): 3875-9.

[68]   Sazuka M, Murakami S, Isemura M, Satoh K, Nukiwa T. Inhibitory effects of green tea infusion on *in vitro* invasion and *in vivo* metastasis of mouse lung carcinoma cells. Cancer Lett 1995; 98(1): 27-31.

[69]   Fu H, He J, Mei F, Zhang Q, Hara Y, Ryota S, *et al.* Lung cancer inhibitory effect of epigallocatechin-3-gallate is dependent on its presence in a complex mixture (polyphenon E). Cancer Prev Res 2009;(6): 531-7.

[70]   Zhang Q, Fu H, Pan J, He J, Ryota S, Hara Y, *et al.* Effect of dietary Polyphenon E and EGCG on lung tumorigenesis in A/J Mice. Pharm Res 2010; 27(6): 1066-71.

[71]   Milligan SA, Burke P, Coleman DT, Bigelow RL, Steffan JJ, Carroll JL, *et al.* The green tea polyphenol EGCG potentiates the antiproliferative activity of c-Met and epidermal growth factor receptor inhibitors in non-small cell lung cancer cells. Clin Cancer Res 2009; 15(15): 4885-94.

[72]   Sadava D, Whitlock E, Kane SE. The green tea polyphenol, epigallocatechin-3-gallate inhibits telomerase and induces apoptosis in drug-resistant lung cancer cells. Biochem Biophys Res Commun 2007; 360(1): 233-7.

[73]   Yang J, Wei D, Liu J. Repressions of MMP-9 expression and NF-kappa B localization are involved in inhibition of lung carcinoma 95-D cell invasion by (-)-epigallocatechin-3-gallate. Biomed Pharmacother 2005; 59(3): 98-103.

[74]   Wu AH, Yu MC, Tseng CC, Hankin J, Pike MC. Green tea and risk of breast cancer in Asian Americans. Int J Cancer 2003; 106(4): 574-9.

[75]   Kumar N, Titus-Ernstoff L, Newcomb PA, Trentham-Dietz A, Anic G, Egan KM. Tea consumption and risk of breast cancer. Cancer Epidemiol Biomarkers Prev 2009; 18(1): 341-5.

[76]   Shrubsole MJ, Lu W, Chen Z, Shu XO, Zheng Y, Dai Q, *et al.* Drinking green tea modestly reduces breast cancer risk. J Nutr 2009; 139(2): 310-6.

[77]   Ogunleye AA, Xue F, Michels KB. Green tea consumption and breast cancer risk or recurrence: a meta-analysis. Breast Cancer Res Treat 2010; 119(2): 477-84.

[78]   Tran PL, Kim SA, Choi HS, Yoon JH, Ahn SG. Epigallocatechin-3-gallate suppresses the expression of HSP70 and HSP90 and exhibits anti-tumor activity *in vitro* and *in vivo.* BMC Cancer 10: 276.

[79]   Sen T, Dutta A, Chatterjee A. Epigallocatechin-3-gallate (EGCG) downregulates gelatinase-B (MMP-9) by involvement of FAK/ERK/NFkappaB and AP-1 in the human breast cancer cell line MDA-MB-231. Anticancer Drugs 2010; 21(6): 632-44.

[80]   Jian L, Lee AH, Binns CW. Tea and lycopene protect against prostate cancer. Asia Pac J Clin Nutr 2007; 16 Suppl 1: 453-7.

[81]   Jian L, Xie LP, Lee AH, Binns CW. Protective effect of green tea against prostate cancer: a case-control study in southeast China. Int J Cancer 2004;108(1): 130-5.

[82]   Kikuchi N, Ohmori K, Shimazu T, Nakaya N, Kuriyama S, Nishino Y, *et al.* No association between green tea and prostate cancer risk in Japanese men: the Ohsaki Cohort Study. Br J Cancer 2006; 95(3): 371-3.

[83]   Brausi M, Rizzi F, Bettuzzi S. Chemoprevention of human prostate cancer by green tea catechins: two years later. A follow-up update. Eur Urol 2008; 54(2): 472-3.

[84]   Bettuzzi S, Brausi M, Rizzi F, Castagnetti G, Peracchia G, Corti A. Chemoprevention of human prostate cancer by oral administration of green tea catechins in volunteers with high-grade prostate intraepithelial neoplasia: a preliminary report from a one-year proof-of-principle study. Cancer Res 2006; 66(2): 1234-40.

[85]   McLarty J, Bigelow RL, Smith M, Elmajian D, Ankem M, Cardelli JA. Tea polyphenols decrease serum levels of prostate-specific antigen, hepatocyte growth factor, and vascular endothelial growth factor in prostate cancer patients and inhibit production of hepatocyte growth factor and vascular endothelial growth factor *in vitro.* Cancer Prev Res 2009; 2(7): 673-82.

[86]   Kurahashi N, Sasazuki S, Iwasaki M, Inoue M, Tsugane S. Green tea consumption and prostate cancer risk in Japanese men: a prospective study. Am J Epidemiol 2008; 167(1): 71-7.

[87]   Adhami VM, Siddiqui IA, Sarfaraz S, Khwaja SI, Hafeez BB, Ahmad N, *et al.* Effective prostate cancer chemopreventive intervention with green tea polyphenols in the TRAMP model depends on the stage of the disease. Clin Cancer Res 2009; 15(6): 1947-53.

[88]   Harper CE, Patel BB, Wang J, Eltoum IA, Lamartiniere CA. Epigallocatechin-3-Gallate suppresses early stage, but not late stage prostate cancer in TRAMP mice: mechanisms of action. Prostate 2007; 67(14): 1576-89.

[89]   Gupta S, Hastak K, Ahmad N, Lewin JS, Mukhtar H. Inhibition of prostate carcinogenesis in TRAMP mice by oral infusion of green tea polyphenols. Proc Natl Acad Sci U S A 2001; 98(18): 10350-5.

[90]   Brusselmans K, De Schrijver E, Heyns W, Verhoeven G, Swinnen JV. Epigallocatechin-3-gallate is a potent natural inhibitor of fatty acid synthase in intact cells and selectively induces apoptosis in prostate cancer cells. Int J Cancer 2003; 106(6): 856-62.

[91]   Hastak K, Gupta S, Ahmad N, Agarwal MK, Agarwal ML, Mukhtar H. Role of p53 and NF-kappaB in epigallocatechin-3-gallate-induced apoptosis of LNCaP cells. Oncogene 2003; 22(31): 4851-9.

[92]   Chuu CP, Chen RY, Kokontis JM, Hiipakka RA, Liao S. Suppression of androgen receptor signaling and prostate specific antigen expression by (-)-epigallocatechin-3-gallate in different progression stages of LNCaP prostate cancer cells. Cancer Lett 2009; 275(1): 86-92.

[93]	Pandey M, Shukla S, Gupta S. Promoter demethylation and chromatin remodeling by green tea polyphenols leads to re-expression of GSTP1 in human prostate cancer cells. Int J Cancer 2010; 126(11): 2520-33.

[94]	Kuo YC, Yu CL, Liu CY, Wang SF, Pan PC, Wu MT, *et al.* A population-based, case-control study of green tea consumption and leukemia risk in southwestern Taiwan. Cancer Causes Control 2009; 20(1): 57-65.

[95]	Zhang M, Zhao X, Zhang X, Holman CD. Possible protective effect of green tea intake on risk of adult leukaemia. Br J Cancer 2008; 98(1): 168-70.

[96]	Naganuma T, Kuriyama S, Kakizaki M, Sone T, Nakaya N, Ohmori-Matsuda K, *et al.* Green tea consumption and hematologic malignancies in Japan: the Ohsaki study. Am J Epidemiol 2009; 170(6): 730-8.

[97]	Shanafelt TD, Lee YK, Call TG, Nowakowski GS, Dingli D, Zent CS, *et al.* Clinical effects of oral green tea extracts in four patients with low grade B-cell malignancies. Leuk Res 2006; 30(6): 707-12.

[98]	Shanafelt TD, Call TG, Zent CS, LaPlant B, Bowen DA, Roos M, *et al.* Phase I trial of daily oral Polyphenon E in patients with asymptomatic Rai stage 0 to II chronic lymphocytic leukemia. J Clin Oncol 2009; 27(23): 3808-14.

[99]	Britschgi A, Simon HU, Tobler A, Fey MF, Tschan MP. Epigallocatechin-3-gallate induces cell death in acute myeloid leukaemia cells and supports all-trans retinoic acid-induced neutrophil differentiation *via* death-associated protein kinase 2. Br J Haematol 2010; 149(1): 55-64.

[100]	Okada N, Tanabe H, Tazoe H, Ishigami Y, Fukutomi R, Yasui K, *et al.* Differentiation-associated alteration in sensitivity to apoptosis induced by (-)-epigallocatechin-3-O-gallate in HL-60 cells. Biomed Res 2009; 30(4): 201-6.

[101]	Han DH, Jeong JH, Kim JH. Anti-proliferative and apoptosis induction activity of green tea polyphenols on human promyelocytic leukemia HL-60 cells. Anticancer Res 2009; 29(4): 1417-21.

[102]	Golden EB, Lam PY, Kardosh A, Gaffney KJ, Cadenas E, Louie SG, *et al.* Green tea polyphenols block the anticancer effects of bortezomib and other boronic acid-based proteasome inhibitors. Blood 2009; 113(23): 5927-37.

[103]	Shah JJ, Kuhn DJ, Orlowski RZ. Bortezomib and EGCG: no green tea for you? Blood 2009; 113(23): 5695-6.

[104]	Wang Q, Li J, Gu J, Huang B, Zhao Y, Zheng D, *et al.* Potentiation of (-)-epigallocatechin-3-gallate-induced apoptosis by bortezomib in multiple myeloma cells. Acta Biochim Biophys Sin (Shanghai) 2009; 41(12): 1018-26.

CHAPTER 5

Receptor Independent Effects of Retinoids

Kinsley Kelley Kiningham[1,*] and Anne Silvis[2]

[1]Department of Pharmaceutical Sciences, Belmont University School of Pharmacy, Gordon E. Inman College of Health Sciences and Nursing, Nashville, TN, USA and [2]Nutrition and Cancer Center, Pharmacology, Physiology and Toxicology, Joan C. Edwards School of Medicine, Marshall University, Huntington, WV, USA

Abstract: Vitamin A, the parent compound of retinoids, was first noted for its role in vision. However, discovery of the ability of retinoids to attenuate tumorigenesis gave rise to a new field of research dedicated to elucidating the mechanisms by which retinoids exhibited antitumor activity. Clinically used since the late 1960's, retinoids comprise a family of structurally similar molecules that exhibit a variety of antitumor effects such as inhibiting cellular proliferation, as well as inducing apoptosis, cell cycle arrest, and differentiation. Much of the early work was strongly focused on signaling pathways influenced by retinoids binding to retinoic acid receptors (RARs). Nonetheless, recent data suggests also receptor-independent mechanisms such as changes in the redox balance within a cell and activation of transcription factors that do not bind the retinoic acid response element. Vitamin A is metabolized into various structural forms such as 9-*cis* retinoic acid (RA), 13-*cis* Retinioc Acid, and all-*trans* Retinioc Acid; additionally, synthetic retinoids have been demonstrated to elicit much of the same effects as the aforementioned endogenous retinoids. Acute promyelocytic leukemia (APL) was one of the first cancers to be successfully treated with 13-*cis* RA. Complications such as toxicity and drug resistance gave rise to clinical trials using all-*trans* Retinioc Acid and, although successful in most patients, a few drug resistant cell populations were discovered. Therefore, decades of research have been aimed to gain a better understanding of both receptor and, most recently, non-receptor mediated signaling pathways which may positively influence future strategies in treatment of various tumors.

Keywords: 13-*cis* Retinoic Acid, Isotretinoin, All-*trans* Retinoic Acid, Cancer, Diet, Differentiation, Food, MnSOD, Nutrition, Reactive Oxygen Species, Retinoic acid, Retinoids, Thiol, Vitamin A.

RETINOIDS

Vitamin A is the parent compound of natural and synthetic retinoid compounds. Retinoids comprise a family of structurally similar molecules (Fig **1**) that exhibit a variety of antitumor effects such as inhibiting cellular proliferation [1], as well as inducing apoptosis [1], cell cycle arrest [2], and differentiation [3]. Retinoids have been used to treat a variety of cancers including acute promyelocytic leukemia (APL) [3], neuroblastoma [3], and cervical dysplasia [4]. Before the 1920's, all of the findings demonstrating the essential nature of vitamin A were focused on its role in vision. Then in 1925, Wolbach and Howe demonstrated that rodents deficient in Vitamin A experienced squamous metaplasia in the trachea and other epithelial sites [5]; reintroduction of Vitamin A reversed this occurrence. In the 1950's and 1960's, Olsen described the metabolism of vitamin A [6] which was followed by recognition of the importance of transport proteins both in the plasma [7] and within the cell [8]. A wave of research ensued in the 1970's and 1980's once Saffiotti *et al.* demonstrated antitumor properties of vitamin A in a lung cancer model [9]. Retinoids were found to exhibit antitumor effects in many animal models such as hamsters [9, 10], mice [11], and rabbits [12]; however, at this time, their effectiveness in humans was still controversial. In particular, all-*trans* retinoic acid (all-*trans* Retinioc Acid, ATRA, tretinoin) and 13-*cis* retinoic acid (13-*cis* Retinioc Acid, isotretinoin) were two of the major metabolites on which most of the research focused. All-*trans* Retinioc Acid is the endogenous ligand synthesized from vitamin A, whereas 13-*cis* Retinioc Acid is a synthetic retinoid that can be isomerized to ATRA (Fig **1**). The effectiveness of both all-*trans*-and 13-*cis* Retinioc Acid as a therapeutic tool for APL was demonstrated in a primary human promyelocytic leukemia cell line (HL-60) [13]. Both of these retinoids could induce differentiation at concentrations much less than previously discovered differentiation-inducing agents.

*Address Correspondence to Kinsley Kelley Kiningham: Department of Pharmaceutical Sciences, Belmont University School of Pharmacy, Gordon E. Inman College of Health Sciences and Nursing, 1900 Belmont Boulevard, Nashville, TN 37212, USA; E-mail: kelley.kiningham@belmont.edu

Pier Paolo Claudio and Richard M. Niles (Eds)

Clinically, APL was initially treated with 13-*cis* Retinioc Acid, and a majority of patients experienced complete remission [14, 15]. However, retinoid use in the clinic has been met with unfavorable outcomes such as toxicity and drug resistance as a result of prolonged treatment [15]. Subsequently, clinical trials with ATRA were initiated and proven to be very effective in many APL patients, where a majority also experienced complete remission. However, a population of APL promyelocytes was isolated from a patient and found *in vitro* to exhibit drug resistance [16]. As a result of these clinical trials, new findings of retinoid receptors were surfacing [17, 18] and scientists learned that such ligand-receptor interactions could either activate or inactivate particular genes. In fact, as will be discussed below, APL is characterized by the prevalence of fusion genes of either the PML or PZLF loci bound to the retinoic acid receptor-alpha (RARα) locus which results in fusion proteins PML-RARα and PZLF-RARα respectively [19, 20]. These receptor-dependent biological effects will be briefly reviewed in this chapter; however, the effects of retinoids (*i.e.* differentiation, apoptosis, growth suppression, drug resistance) need to be further evaluated in light of recent findings suggesting that non-receptor mediated events are initiated in multiple cell types as a result of exposure to both synthetic and naturally occurring retinoids.

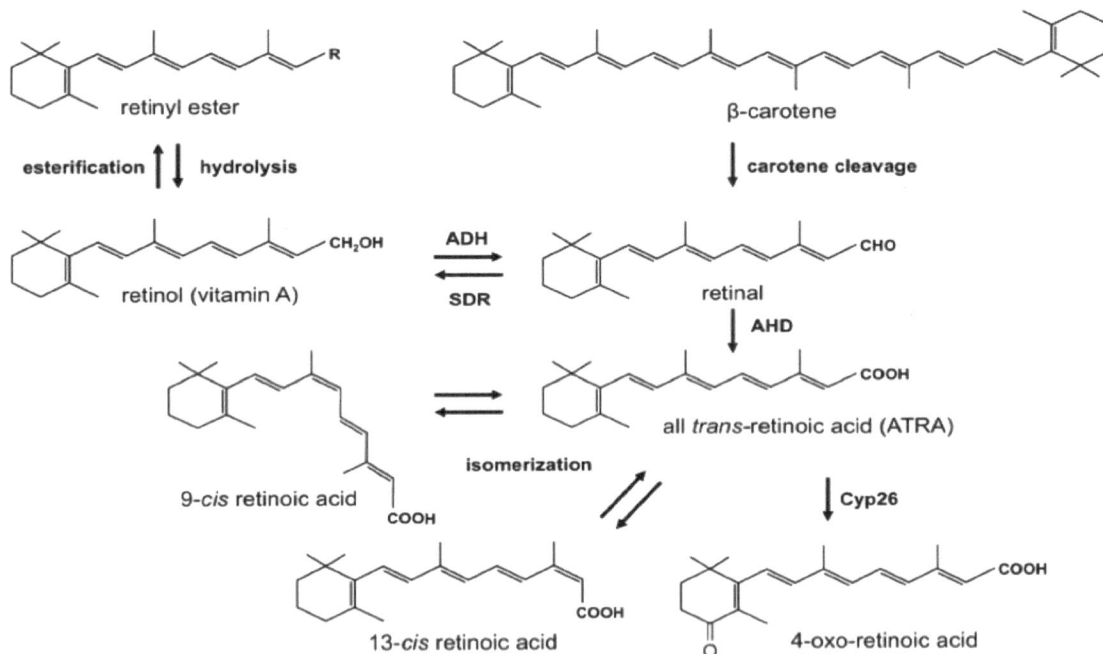

Figure 1: Naturally occurring retinoids. β-carotene, found in plant-derived foods, is cleaved to form two molecules of retinal. Retinyl esters (R: fatty acid), found in animal-derived foods, are hydrolyzed to retiniol. Retinol is reversibly converted to retinal by alcohol dehydrogenase (ADH). Retinal is irreversibly converted to ATRA *via* aldehyide dehydrogenase (ADH). ATRA can be isomerized into 9-*cis* retinoic acid or 13-*cis* retinoic acid. ATRA can also be irreversibly oxidized to form metabolites such as 4-oxo-retinoic acid by cytochrome P450 Cyp16. SDR, short-chain dehydrogenase.

RETINOID METABOLISM

Not only is vitamin A metabolized into various structural forms, but there is much evidence to show that synthetic retinoids (Fig **2**) can elicit similar effects as endogenous retinoids. Furthermore, in any respective study, there is often debate as to which metabolite is biologically active, *i.e.* the one to which cellular effects can be ascribed. Therefore, it is essential to critically review the current literature in light of these aspects.

Vitamin A cannot be synthesized endogenously, but must be obtained in our diet. Animal-derived foods contain preformed vitamin A that is predominantly in the form of retinyl esters; whereas plant-derived foods contain pro-vitamin A carotenoids, such as β-carotene (reviewed in [21, 22] (Fig **1**). A majority of this pro-and preformed vitamin A is converted to all-*trans* retinol (vitamin A) by a series of reactions that occur in the intestinal lumen and mucosa. Retinol can be re-esterified after absorption by enterocytes and then packaged into chylomicrons for transportation to and storage in the liver. According to the body's needs, these retinyl esters are re-hydrolyzed to retinol, which is secreted from the liver bound to retinol binding protein (RBP). Once retinol reaches its target cell, it can be handled in a variety of ways. Its lipophilic nature allows it to freely diffuse across cellular membranes; or bound with RBP, it may signal through the cell surface receptor Stra6 [23]. Retinol can then be reversibly converted to retinal by alcohol dehydrogenase (ADH), which is then irreversibly converted to the bioactive form ATRA *via* aldehyde dehydrogenase (AHD). All-*trans* Retinioc Acid can either be 1) metabolized into other forms such as the 9-*cis* retinoic acid and 13-*cis* retinoic acid isomers or 4-oxo-retinoic acid, or 2) translocated by cellular retinoic acid binding proteins (CRABP-I, -II) to the nucleus for binding to nuclear receptors. All-*trans* Retinioc Acid is the most potent and the main signaling retinoid *in vivo*. Not only has it been very effective to treat APL [3], but it is also used to battle other cancers including neuroblastoma [3], and medulloblastoma [24]. Metabolism (*i.e.* double-bond isomerization and oxidation) of endogenous retinoids can sometimes result in deleterious effects such as a decrease in activity and selectivity. Therefore, scientists have attempted to overcome these limitations by constructing synthetic retinoids which are often more stable and more active [22] (Fig **2**).

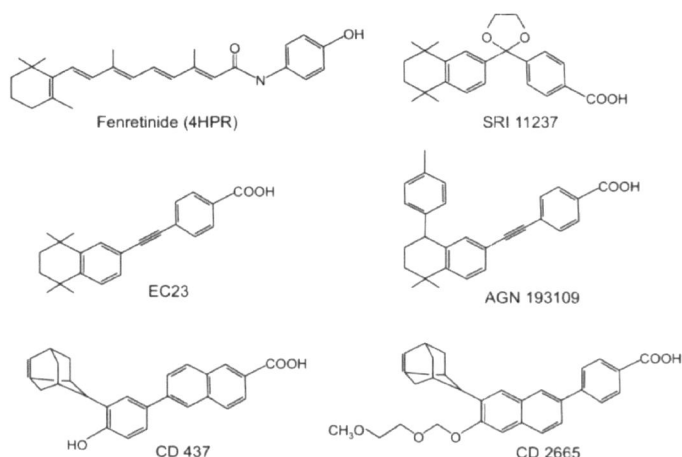

Figure 2: Structures of synthetic retinoids. Retinoids agonists: Fenretinide, EC23, CD 437; rexinoid agonist: SRI 11237; RAR antagonist: AGN 193109, CD 2665.

Most work to date has focused on retinoid-mediated gene regulation through the nuclear retinoic acid receptors; however, there are reports to suggest some retinoid effects to be a result of receptor-independent mechanisms. It must also be considered that any such action of retinoids can be the result of activation of both pathways.

RETINOID MECHANISM OF ACTION

The biological actions of retinoids are mediated in part by heterodimerization of nuclear retinoic acid receptors (RAR-α, -β, and-γ) and retinoid "X" receptors (RXR-α, -β, and-γ). Each subtype of the receptors is encoded for by different genes that have multiple promoters, and each gene product can undergo differential splicing. Therefore, the array of isoforms that exist between RARs and RXRs gives rise to numerous combinations of receptor dimerizations [21]. The ligand specificities of these receptors differ. All-*trans*-and 9-*cis*-RA can bind to the RARs, but RXRs only bind 9-*cis*-RA [25, 26] (Fig **3**). Affinities for various receptors differ also in the fact that RARs bind ATRA with higher affinity than 9-*cis* Retinioc Acid [27]. The metabolite 13-*cis* Retinioc Acid can either bind to RAR in its native configuration [28], or bind in the form of ATRA after isomerization [29]. Once bound by a ligand, the RAR-RXR heterodimer binds to the retinoic acid response element (RARE); whereas RXR homodimers bind to RXREs [27]. It is worth noting that retinoic acid can bind with high affinity to another receptor (peroxisome proliferator-activated receptors, PPARβ/γ) [30], which also functions as a heterodimer with RXR [31]. RXR-PPAR heterodimers bind as a complex to the peroxisome proliferator response element (PPRE). ATRA binding to PPAR receptors has been suggested to promote cell survival [32] and to mediate retinoic acid resistance [33]. Retinoic acid response elements are contained within the regulatory regions of numerous genes involved in retinoid signaling; however, retinoids can indirectly regulate a number of genes that are targets of regulatory proteins (such as transcription factors) whose expression is directly regulated by activated RAR/RXR; these secondary genes do not possess a RARE. All-*trans* Retinioc Acid can also exhibit non-receptor mediated effects such as changes in redox balance within a cell [34] or activation of transcription factors that do not bind the RARE [35, 36]. It is these receptor-independent mechanisms that will be discussed in further detail regarding the therapeutic use of retinoids in various cancer models.

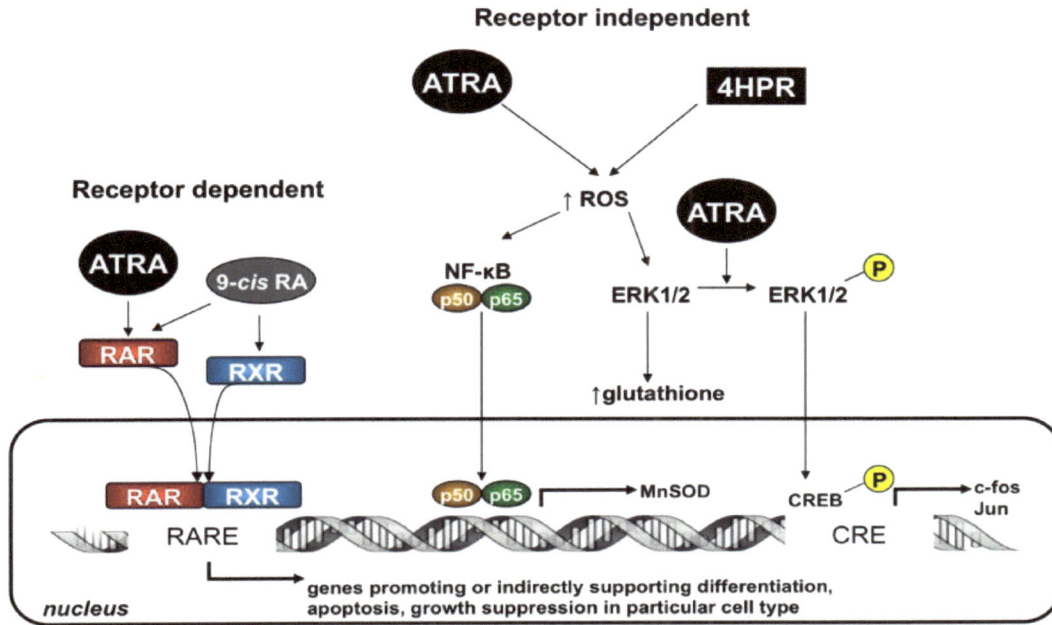

Figure 3: Retinoid mechanism of action. Retinoid acid (RA) can modulate gene expression to promote differentiation, apoptosis, or growth suppression *via* receptor-dependent or –independent mechanism. ATRA: All-*trans* retinoic acid; 9-*cis* Retinioc Acid: 9-*cis* retinoic acid; 4HPR: Fenretinide; ROS: Reactive oxygen species.

The common means by which retinoids are known to antagonize carcinogenesis are either by inducing differentiation and apoptosis and/or suppressing proliferation. Current research efforts are devoted to identifying the exact mechanisms by which retinoids accomplish these actions. Moreover, there is a vast difference amongst studies regarding the type of retinoids (natural *vs.* synthetic), concentration (micromolar range), the duration of treatment (days to weeks), and the particular model (*in vitro, in vivo, ex vivo*). Various cancers have a particular sensitivity to any one of the retinoids. For example, 9-*cis* Retinioc Acid is a very effective differentiation agent for neuroblastoma cells *in vitro* [37, 38], however the toxicity of 9-*cis* Retinioc Acid *in vivo* may limit its clinical potential [39]. Cells experience much less toxicity with ATRA; however, its effectiveness has been limited by a short half-life and decreased plasma levels due to drug metabolism [3]. Nonetheless, scientists have been dedicated to optimizing retinoid therapy in ways such as decreasing toxic side effects [40], increasing bioavailability [41, 42], and enhancing effectiveness by co-administration of other agents [43, 44].

RETINOIDS AND REACTIVE OXYGEN SPECIES (ROS)

Retinoids have also been demonstrated to alter the levels of ROS in various cancer models. Interestingly, ROS represent a biological paradox. They are essential to prevent disease by initiating signaling cascades (*i.e.*) to promote apoptosis; however, increased levels have the potential to damage important macromolecules and thus may play a role in promoting carcinogenesis [45]. Reactive oxygen species are generated naturally in the cell primarily by means of the electron transport chain. Nearly 1-3% of oxygen consumed by the body is converted into ROS; three of the most prominent being superoxide radical, hydrogen peroxide and hydroxyl radical.

Therefore, cells have developed a means to keep the levels of ROS in check to avoid the events of carcinogenesis. Such a response involves the presence of antioxidants: some of which are enzymatic (superoxide dismutases, catalase, and glutathione peroxidase) and others of which are non-enzymatic (glutathione, thiols, vitamins).

One broad class of molecules that ROS can influence is the mitogen-activated protein kinases (MAPKs). For example, extracellular regulated kinase [29] activation is typically associated with cell survival in response to ROS [46]; however, ERK can also promote apoptosis in certain cell types including human leukemia U937 cells [47]. This disparity may be explained by the method of ERK activation; rapid and transient versus slow and sustained. It may also be explained by the endogenous levels of antioxidants as these can affect the levels of ROS experienced by the cells. The ubiquitously expressed mammalian transcription factor nuclear factor kappa B (NF-κB) is activated in response to numerous stimuli, including ROS, and has been reported to play roles in the differentiation of both APL and neuroblastoma [48-50]. Reactive oxygen species are also known to modulate the immune response; for example, by stimulating synthesis of pro-inflammatory cytokines [51]. Early studies by Rudolf Virchow in 1863 [52] suggested that chronic inflammation is a major factor in promoting carcinogenesis since. Virchow recognized the presence of leukocytes in neoplastic tissues; and since this observation, there has been a multitude of supporting data identifying the origination of tumors at sites of chronic inflammation [53]. In fact, chronic infections and inflammations contribute to as much as 25% of global cancer cases [54].

As will be discussed in more detail below, retinoids mediate some of their effects *via* enhancing the generation of ROS. For example, ATRA induced apoptosis and increased peroxide generation within 24 hours of *in vitro* exposure to acute myeloblastic leukemia (AML) cells [34]. Gelain *et al.* report that retinol, not retinoic acid, increased ROS in PC12 cells, a model system for primary neurons [55]. Fenretinide (N-(4-Hydroxyphenyl)retinamide; 4HPR) is a synthetic retinoid that classically promotes apoptosis *via* non-receptor dependent mechanisms that generate ROS [3, 56, 57]. However, there is evidence to suggest its effects may also involve receptor activation [58]. The redox status of a cell (determined by the balance of ROS and antioxidants) can influence and regulate a multitude of cellular processes including proliferation, differentiation, and death [34, 59, 60]. Given the numerous studies demonstrating that retinoids influence ROS formation, it is apparent that the alteration of redox status by retinoids likely contributes to the modulation of genes which are Involved In Cellular Processes Such As Differentiation, Apoptosis, And/Or Chemoresistance.

RETINOIDS EFFECTS ON DIFFERENTIATION

Acute promyelocytic leukemia is the original and most widely studied cancer model by which differentiation therapy with ATRA is used [16, 61]. It is characterized by the prevalence of a fusion protein (PML-RARα) due to a t(15;17) chromosomal translocation [19, 20]. It is generally accepted that this PML-RARα fusion protein generates a differentiation block such that RARα is unable to transcriptionally regulate essential genes involved in differentiation when heterodimerizing with RXR. Historically, ATRA therapy is believed to induce promyelocytic differentiation by degradation of the PML-RARα fusion protein *via* binding to its receptors [62]. However, there is evidence to suggest that ATRA can also induce APL cells to differentiate in a RAR-independent manner [63]. The alternate differentiation response may involve cross-talk between RXR agonists and protein kinase A [64]. *In vitro* studies demonstrated that full maturation of NB4 cells (ATRA-responsive cells derived from an APL patient) was achieved in the presence of a rexinoid agonist (SRI 11237), which does not induce RAR activity, in combination with a cyclic AMP-dependent protein kinase [64] agonist (8CPT-cAMP). Such maturation was not observed in the presence of either agonist when administered alone. Therefore, signaling activity mediated by the RAR was not essential for ATRA-induced granulocytic differentiation.

There is evidence to support the possibility of either a retinoid-mediated increase or a decrease in ROS as a mechanism for differentiation. This paradox might be due to the experimental model, species or concentration of retinoid used, and even the duration of treatment. However, there are few studies that investigate these mechanisms in cancer cells. One study focuses on myeloid derived suppressor cells (MDSCs), which are produced in large numbers in patients having a variety of different cancers [65]. These cells are relatively immature cells and have characteristically high ROS production. This ROS production 1) promotes MDSC-mediated T-cell suppression and 2) contributes to the inability of MDSCs to differentiate [66, 67]. Since ATRA has been shown to effectively differentiate these cells in culture, ATRA is believed to be a valuable tool for cancer immunotherapy in such a model. The mechanism by which ATRA differentiated MDSCs was suggested to be in part *via* upregulation of glutathione (GSH) synthesis and the downregulation of ROS [65]. Glutathione is the predominant non-protein thiol in the cell and is perhaps the most essential factor in maintaining cellular redox homeostasis [68]. It is important to note that in these experiments, a short exposure (48 hours) with relatively low concentrations of ATRA (1.5 µM) was used to these cells. Furthermore, the ability of ATRA to increase protein expression of glutathione synthase (GS, a GSH synthesizing enzyme) was not a result of any RAR activity; *i.e.* there was no direct binding of an RAR in the GS promoter. Rather there was a concomitant increase in ERK 1/2 activation, which was suggested to play a role in regulating GS protein expression.

On the other hand, retinoids have been reported to generate ROS in both patient APL cell types and the human promyelocytic leukemia cell line (HL-60). Leukocytes characteristically produce ROS, in particular superoxide, which has been correlated with differentiation [69, 70]. Thus, differentiation is determined by PMA-induced superoxide production and cytoplasmic superoxide is assayed by its ability to reduce soluble NBT (nitroblue tetrazolium) to a blue-black precipitate, formazan. P19 embryonal carcinoma cells have also been used as a model of retinoid induced differentiation and to demonstrate the importance of ROS in neuronal differentiation [64]. Retinoic acid-induced differentiation was coupled with increased ROS production, which was evaluated by the use of dihydrorhodamine, an indicator of peroxynitrite formation [71]. Under serum-free conditions, P19 cells were cultured in the presence of Retinioc Acid (unknown species) also at very low concentrations (0.2 µM) only for 1 hour prior to addition of scavengers of ROS. These scavengers, including glutathione, N-acetyl-L-cysteine, and ascorbic acid, not only reduced expression of differentiation markers, but also attenuated Retinioc Acid-induced activity of the RARE. Therefore, these studies suggest that RAR receptor activity played an integral part to promote differentiation that was dependent on an increase in ROS in this cell type. However, no direct link was demonstrated. In considering these varying results, we suggest that whether an increase or decrease in ROS contributes to differentiation, depends on the cell types studied, their baseline redox state and their endogenous levels and types of antioxidants.

Not only have retinoids been proven effective against APL, but clinical trials within the past decade have demonstrated successful treatment of juvenile malignancies such as neuroblastoma [72]. Neuroblastoma is the most common extracranial solid tumor in childhood, representing 7-10% of all pediatric cancers. A number of retinoids have been used in clinical trials to fight this childhood cancer including 13-*cis* Retinioc Acid, 9-*cis* Retinioc Acid, ATRA, and synthetic homologues such as fenretinide [3]. A recent finding demonstrated that ATRA-induced differentiation of neuroblastoma cells lead to nuclear accumulation of p27 *via* destabilization of Skp2, an E3 ubiquitin ligase SCF activator, which targeted p27 for degradation [73]. A cyclin dependent kinase (CDK) inhibitor, p27 is a negative regulator of cellular proliferation. Therefore, accumulation of p27 in the nucleus would result in a halt of the cell cycle, which likely permits the cell to undergo differentiation. In mammalian cells, antimitogenic factors cause cell cycle arrest in the G_1 phase, and differentiation (aside from senescence) is typically associated with cell cycle withdrawal in the presence of such factors. Therefore, agents that induce growth arrest can have the potential to also induce differentiation [74]. The mechanism by which ATRA promoted Skp2 destabilization in the aforementioned studies was through the activation of the anaphase promoting complex (APC^{Cdh1}), a member of the ubiquitin ligase family. Interestingly, this study highlights two key pathways being regulated by ATRA; the cell-cycle and the proteasome ubiquitin system. Retinoids also alter transcriptional expression of genes involved in proliferation arrest and cell cycle exit in numerous cell lines representing different types of tumors. Exposure of the myelomonoblastic cell line U937 to ATRA resulted in growth arrest and a simultaneous upregulation of the CDK inhibitor p21 [75]. Not surprisingly, protein and mRNA levels and activity of p21 increased prior to differentiation of these cells into monocytes.

Moreover, retinoid-induced differentiation in this model was mediated *via* retinoid receptor activity as a RAR-RXR heterodimer has been demonstrated to be bound to an RARE within the p21 gene. As mentioned above, the ubiquitin degradation system can also be regulated by retinoids. Retinoids can induce degradation of cyclin D1, an important regulator of cell cycle progression that is either overexpressed or deregulated in several types of cancers [76, 77]. These findings are supported by studies demonstrating degradation of PML-RARα in ATRA-mediated differentiation of APL [78-80]. The degradation of PML-RARα has been suggested to be due to both the proteasome-ubiquitin and the caspase systems [81]. In APL cells, the addition of caspase inhibitors significantly blocked Retinoic Acid-mediated PML-RARα degradation; and recombinant caspases (1, 6, and 7) were capable of cleaving PML. Subsequent experiments were performed in the presence of a caspase inhibitor (z-VAD), etoposide (an activator of caspases) or both compounds. Treatment with etoposide resulted in the disappearance of full-size PML and the caspase inhibitor restored PML expression, demonstrating that PML is a target of caspase.

NF-κB has been reported to play important roles in the differentiation of both APL and neuroblastoma [48-50]. One study reported that synergy between ATRA and tumor necrosis factor (TNF) is a mechanism for enhancing differentiation of APL cells [48]. Using an NF-κB reporter construct, ATRA alone strongly stimulated NF-κB activity (10.8-fold) whereas TNF alone had only a modest induction of activity (1.8-fold). However, in concert, the two synergistically induced NF-κB activity 24-fold compared with untreated cells. In parallel, there was a significant enhancement of monocyte differentiation markers. Furthermore, analysis of RAR regulated pathways revealed that TNF did not enhance transcription of RAR targeted genes (*i.e.* RARβ, C/EBP epsilon) over that of ATRA alone. This study suggests that TNF works by a retinoid receptor receptor-independent mechanism to enhance ATRA-mediated differentiation of APL cells *via* NF-κB activation. In contrast, another study investigating the role of NF-κB in ATRA-induced maturation of this same cell type (NB4 cells), used the same concentration (1 μM) of ATRA, but the duration of treatment was slightly longer. This group discovered that inhibition of NF-κB transcriptional activity did not impede differentiation and concluded that NF-κB was not essential for retinoid-induced differentiation in this cell line. Another recent study utilized the SK-N-SH neuroblastoma cell line to demonstrate that NF-κB activation was necessary for ATRA-mediated neuronal differentiation [49].

Furthermore, the studies also suggested that ATRA induces the expression of manganese superoxide dismutase (MnSOD) *via* the activation of NF-κB. Manganese superoxide dismutase is a mitochondrial enzyme that is upregulated in response to ROS generation and converts the superoxide anion to hydrogen peroxide and molecular oxygen [82, 83]. Since MnSOD activity was increased in comparison to the undifferentiated progenitors [84], it has also been suggested to play a role in the process of cellular differentiation in human monocytes [85], rat embryo fibroblasts [86], and neuroblastoma cells, Use of an NF-κB inhibitor peptide attenuated ATRA-mediated expression of MnSOD [49]. Therefore, ATRA did not directly activate a component of the MnSOD gene by binding a RAR/RXR; however, these data do not rule out that this was a secondary effect. It has yet to be established whether ATRA upregulated NF-κB *via* retinoid receptor activity, which then could have been bound to the MnSOD gene. As stated above, basal or induced expression of antioxidants are important to consider in any cellular response, especially those involving NF-κB, since this transcription factor is commonly upregulated in response to an increase in ROS.

Evidence is mounting to demonstrate that retinoid-induced differentiation can also modulate rapid kinase signaling pathways by mechanisms independent of receptor binding [87, 88]. The transcription factor cAMP response element binding protein (CREB) is a major downstream effector of ERK1/2 signaling that contributes to differentiation in many cellular models [89, 90]. In a subclone of PC12 neuronal cells Retinoic Acid-induced phosphorylation of CREB resulted in activation of early genes such as c-jun and c-fos, which do not contain RARE's, and are suggested to play a role in mediating neuronal differentiation of PC12 cells [87]. Furthermore, they demonstrated that ERK activation was essential for the observed CREB phosphorylation. Other groups confirmed these findings in human bronchial epithelial cells and additionally identified a receptor-independent mechanism by demonstrating that silencing RAR/RXR expression did not affect Retinoic Acid's ability to increase the phosphorylation of CREB [88].

RETINOIDS EFFECTS ON PROLIFERATION AND APOPTOSIS

Retinoids are well established as inducers of apoptosis or suppressors of proliferation in several tumor models. Another well studied model of retinoid-induced growth arrest and differentiation is the F9 murine embryonal carcinoma cell line. These cells resemble the pluripotent stem cells in the early mouse embryo that differentiate into any of the three endodermal cell types (primitive, parietal, and visceral) in the presence of ATRA. In addition, under the certain conditions retinoids can also induce growth suppression and apoptosis in these cells [91, 92]. A series of F9 cell lines null for expression of RARα, RARγ, RXRα, and combinations of RARα-RXRα and RARγ-RXRα were generated in order to delineate the functional importance of RAR and RXR [92-95]. Investigators provided evidence for the receptor-dependent differential requirements of RARs and RXR in mediating retinoid-induced cellular differentiation, proliferation, and death of the F9 embryonal carcinoma cells [96]. However, the ability of the synthetic retinoid Fenretinide to induce apoptosis in cells that are resistant to ATRA suggested receptor-independent functions of retinoid therapy in certain cell types [56, 97, 98]. Therefore, Clifford *et al.* subjected the mutant F9 cells that lack RARγ, RXRα, or both proteins, to treatment with either Fenretinide (10 μM) or ATRA (10 μM) [99]. Cellular viability assays demonstrated that within 48 hours, Fenretinide decreased viability in all receptor-null cell lines to levels similar to those of the F9 wild type (WT) cell line. This loss of cellular viability was confirmed to be a combination of apoptosis and necrosis, as determined by Hoechst 3328 and PI (propidium iodide) staining respectively. Comparable studies done with ATRA showed a minimal loss of viability after 48 hours. Furthermore, extended treatments (4-5 days) with ATRA resulted in differentiation, growth suppression, and apoptosis in F9 WT but not in receptor-null cells. This suggested that the delayed effects of ATRA were receptor-dependent and distinct from the rapid receptor-independent reduction in cellular viability elicited by Fenretinide. Interestingly, at lower concentrations, Fenretinide (1 μM) induced differentiation resembling that of ATRA (1μM) treatment of F9 WT cell lines but not in the RARγ/RXRα knockout (KO) lines, suggesting that the latter effects are likely due to the presence of receptors. As noted by the authors, a potential mechanism for Fenretinide-induced cellular death may have been *via* the generation of ROS.

Evidence supporting this hypothesis stems from studies showing that the antioxidants vitamin E and N-acetyl-L-cysteine inhibited Fenretinide-induced apoptosis in human HL-60 leukemia cells [100]. Furthermore, other studies have demonstrated that retinoid-induced apoptosis in cervical carcinoma cells coincided with ROS production as measured by the oxidation-sensitive fluorescent dye 5, 6-carboxy-28, 78-dicholorfluorescin diacetate (DCFH-DA) [57]. DCFH-DA fluoresces not only in the presence of hydrogen peroxide, but also other ROS such as peroxynitrite [101]. Addition of the antioxidant pyrrolidine dithiocarbamate (PDTC, a thiol antioxidant and metal chelating compound) reversed the Fenretinide-induced apoptotic process. Fenretinide (0.08-10 μM) increased the levels of ROS in as early as 20 minutes; whereas no such induction was observed in the presence of ATRA (0.1-10 μM) or the retinoid agonist CD437 (0.1-1 μM) [57]. Although Fenretinide did not bind to retinoid receptors in this study, it reportedly did induce transactivation of the RARE (data was not shown). However, considering that ATRA did not induce apoptosis of these cells and that the RAR antagonist CD2665 did not inhibit Fenretinide's effects on cellular viability, it is unlikely that these effects were RAR receptor-mediated. Instead, it is likely that Fenretinide-induced apoptosis in this model involved cross-talk between RXR agonists and other signaling pathways (PKA, MAPK, *etc.*) to activate the RARE independent of RAR receptors. This is supported by studies performed by Benoit *et al.* [63] demonstrating cross-talk between RXR agonists and protein kinase A [64] in ATRA-mediated differentiation of APL cells.

Retinoids have been reported to generate ROS, particularly superoxide, in APL, an effect that is coupled with suppressed growth and apoptosis [34]. These studies utilized two different human acute myeloblastic leukemia (AML) cell lines that differ in their responsiveness to ATRA; ATRA-sensitive OU-AML-3 and ATRA-resistant OU-AML-7. ATRA-mediated growth suppression and apoptosis (Annexin V positive cells) after 72 hours of treatment was more prominent in OU-AML-3 cells than the OU-AML-7 cells. Furthermore, these decreases were preceded by an increase in ROS (DCFH-DA) at 24 hours. Interestingly, ATRA was also shown to promote antioxidant properties in these cells by increasing γ-glutamylcysteine synthetase (γ-GCS) activity and expression of MnSOD, again to a greater degree in the ATRA-sensitive OU-AML-3 cells. As the rate-limiting enzyme in glutathione synthesis, γ-GCS plays an essential role to increase glutathione content in cells. High γ-GCS and glutathione levels have both been shown to be associated with increased resistance in many cancer models [102, 103].

As mentioned earlier, retinoid-induced differentiation in APL is associated with PML-RARα degradation. Interestingly, the degradation of PML-RARα and the release of PML have been demonstrated to lead cells to apoptosis [104, 105]. Although PML-RARα is degraded 12–24 hours after application of ATRA in APL cells, apoptosis does not occur until after terminal differentiation [62]. Moreover, gene expression analysis revealed that the balance between apoptosis and differentiation could be maintained through the induction of anti-apoptotic molecules and the inhibition of apoptosis agonists.

In recent years, there has been much focus on utilizing retinoid therapy as a means of treatment for melanoma [106]. With a high mortality rate, the incidence of metastatic melanoma has been steadily increasing within the past three decades [107]. If diagnosed early, surgical removal is a highly successful option. However, once it reaches advanced stages, melanoma is substantially resistant to radio-and chemotherapy. Because patients respond differently to retinoid treatment, there are many cell lines that are used to model the disease; some of which are resistant to the effects of Retinioc Acid and those of which are not. Retinoic acid slows the replication of the S91 murine melanoma cells by repression of genes involved in proliferation and cell division, which precedes differentiation [108]. This study also demonstrates that in the presence of Retinioc Acid, cellular viability remained intact and differentiation was receptor-mediated and exclusively dependent on expression of RARγ. Quite interestingly, the RARγ-specific agonist CD437 (6-(3-(1-adamantyl)-4-hydroxyphenyl)-2-naphthoic acid, AHPN) can not only induce differentiation of these cells, but also apoptosis thereafter within 8 hours [109]. Furthermore, it has also been reported that 1) CD347 promoted apoptosis in Retinioc Acid-resistant cells and 2) RAR-antagonists could not block CD437-mediated apoptosis. Therefore, it is apparent that this RARγ agonist can elicit receptor-independent mechanisms to induce apoptosis in melanoma cells. Zhao *et al.* discovered five genes that were differentially upregulated in CD437 *vs.* Retinioc Acid-treated murine S91 cells treated for 8 hours with 1 μM) of the retinoid (p21, MDM2, TEAP, cyclin G1, and ei24). In previously described studies ATRA upregulated p21 expression in the U937 myelomonoblastic cell line; however, this is a completely different model cell line/tumor, and different retinoid concentrations (0.1 μM) were administered for a different amount of time (72 hours).

Retinoids have also been proven to be very effective to inhibit colon cancer cell growth [110, 111] and earlier work indicates that low retinol levels may contribute to increased risk for recurrence of colorectal cancer [112]. A recent study demonstrated that the ability of retinol to inhibit growth in ATRA-resistant colon cancer cell lines was RAR-independent [111]. Retinol (vitamin A) is the parent compound, of which ATRA is a biologically active metabolite; therefore, metabolism of retinol was initially assessed to ascertain which species of retinol metabolite was responsible for these effects. In both ATRA-sensitive and ATRA-resistant colon cancer cells, there was little to no production of ATRA or other retinol metabolites such as 2-oxoretinol or anhydroretinol during a 96 hour incubation with retinol (upon which suppression of growth was observed). A RARE-CAT (chloramphenicol acetyltransferase) vector harboring the regulatory region of RARβ2 was constructed to assess retinoid binding to the RARE. The inability of retinol to induce CAT activity in the ATRA-sensitive cells reflected its inability to be metabolized into ATRA. Furthermore, neither ATRA nor retinol induced CAT activity in any of the ATRA-resistant cell lines, despite the conversion of retinol into ATRA, albeit very low. Therefore, in all model cell types, retinol elicited its effects in a manner independent of, at least, the RARβ2 receptor. The inability of the RAR pan antagonist AGN 193109 to block retinol-induced growth inhibition confirmed these conclusions. Moreover, retinol did not induce apoptosis, differentiation, or necrosis within 96 hours in any of the ATRA-resistant cell lines, indicating in these models that retinol does not inhibit colon cancer cell growth *via* promoting apoptosis. The same group has recently followed up this study with one demonstrating retinol-mediated inhibition of colon cancer cell invasion *via* a decrease matrix metalloproteinase activity [113].

CONCLUSIONS

The ability of both natural and synthetic retinoids to induce processes such as differentiation, apoptosis, and growth suppression in cancer cells has been extensively studied. Although a significant amount of research to date has focused on RAR-dependent effects, there is increasing evidence for mechanisms independent of the receptor (see Table 1). Among these are generation/reduction of ROS, which can result in the activation of transcription factors such as NF-κB or CREB; activation of RXR pathways independent of the RAR; activation of MAPK pathways; initiation of proteasomal degradation pathways; and inhibition of cell cycle components. A more complete understanding of these receptor–independent mechanisms is essential in order to enhance the effectiveness of retinoids and to avoid the occurrence of chemoresistance.

Table 1: Receptor-independent effects of particular retinoids

Retinoid	Mechanism	Effect	Reference
ATRA	↑ ROS	Cell growth inhibition, Apoptosis	Mantymaa, Guttorn *et al.* 2000 [34]
	↓ ROS (↑ GSH)	Differentiation	Nefedova, Fishman *et al.* 2007 [65]
	↑ p27	Differentiation	Cuende, Moreno *et al.* 2008 [73]
	↑ p21	Growth Arrest	Liu, Lavarone *et al.* 1996 [5]
	↑ proteasome/caspases	Differentiation	Zhu, Gianni *et al.* 1999 [81]
	↑ NF-κB/TNF	Differentiation	Witcher, Ross *et al.* 2003; Kiningham, Cardozo *et al.* 2008 [48, 49]
	↑ MnSOD	Differentiation	Kiningham, Cardozo *et al.* 2008 [49]
Retinol	↑ ROS	Apoptosis	Gelain and Moreira 2008
	?	Cell growth Inhibition Decrease invasion	Park, Dillard *et al.* 2005
	↓ MMP		Park, Wilder *et al.* 2007
Retinoic Acid (isotype NA)	↑ ROS	Differentiation	Konopka, Kubala *et al.* 2008; Crow *et al.* 1997
	p-CREB (*c-jun, c-fos*)	Differentiation	Canon, Cosgaya *et al.* 2004
Fenretinide	↑ ROS	Apoptosis	Reynolds and Lemons 2001; Delia *et al.* 1993; Oridate, Suzuki *et al.* 1997; Clifford, Menter *et al.* 1999 [3, 56, 57, 99]
SRI 11237 (rexinoid agonist)	RXR/PKA	Differentiation	Benoit, Altucci *et al.* 1999 [63]
CD 437 (RARγ-agonist)	p21, MDM2	Apoptosis	Zhao, Demary *et al.* 2001 [109]

REFERENCES

[1]   Altucci L, Gronemeyer H. The promise of retinoids to fight against cancer. Nat Rev Cancer 2001; 1(3): 181-93.

[2]   Donato LJ, Suh JH, Noy N. Suppression of mammary carcinoma cell growth by retinoic acid: the cell cycle control gene Btg2 is a direct target for retinoic acid receptor signaling. Cancer Res 2007; 67(2): 609-15.

[3]   Reynolds CP, Lemons RS. Retinoid therapy of childhood cancer. Hematol Oncol Clin North Am 2001; 15(5): 867-910.

[4]   Meyskens FL, Jr., Surwit E, Moon TE, *et al.* Enhancement of regression of cervical intraepithelial neoplasia II (moderate dysplasia) with topically applied all-*trans*-retinoic acid: a randomized trial. J Natl Cancer Inst 1994; 86(7): 539-43.

[5]   Wolbach SB, Howe PR. Nutrition Classics. The Journal of Experimental Medicine 42: 753-77, 1925. Tissue changes following deprivation of fat-soluble A vitamin. S. Burt Wolbach and Percy R. Howe. Nutr Rev 1978; 36(1): 16-9.

[6]   Blaner WS, Olson JA. Retinol and retinoic acid metabolism. In: Sporn MB, Roberts, A.B., Goodman, D.S., editor. The Retinoids, 2nd Ed New York: Raven Press; 1994. p. 229-56.

[7]   Goodman DS. Plasma retinol-binding protein. Sporn MB, Roberts, A.B., Goodman, D.S., editor. New York: Academic Press; 1984.

[8]   Ong DD, Newcomer ME, Chytil F. Cellular retinoid-binding proteins. Sporn MB, Roberts, A.B., Goodman, D.S., editor. New York: Raven Press; 1994.

[9]   Saffiotti U, Montesano R, Sellakumar AR, Borg SA. Experimental cancer of the lung. Inhibition by vitamin A of the induction of tracheobronchial squamous metaplasia and squamous cell tumors. Cancer 1967; 20(5): 857-64.

[10]   Chu EW, Malmgren RA. An inhibitory effect of vitamin A on the induction of tumors of forestomach and cervix in the Syrian hamster by carcinogenic polycyclic hydrocarbons. Cancer Res 1965; 25(6): 884-95.

[11]   Davies RE. Effect of vitamin A on 7,12-Dimethylbenz(alpha)anthracene-induced papillomas in rhino mouse skin. Cancer Res 1967; 27(2): 237-41.

[12]   McMichael H. Inhibition of growth of Shope rabbit papilloma by hypervitaminosis A. Cancer Res 1965; 25(7): 947-55.

[13]   Breitman TR, Selonick SE, Collins SJ. Induction of differentiation of the human promyelocytic leukemia cell line (HL-60) by retinoic acid. Proc Natl Acad Sci U S A 1980; 77(5): 2936-40.

[14]   Daenen S, Vellenga E, van Dobbenburgh OA, Halie MR. Retinoic acid as antileukemic therapy in a patient with acute promyelocytic leukemia and Aspergillus pneumonia. Blood 1986; 67(2): 559-61.

[15]   Fontana JA, Rogers JS, 2nd, Durham JP. The role of 13 cis-retinoic acid in the remission induction of a patient with acute promyelocytic leukemia. Cancer 1986; 57(2): 209-17.

[16]   Huang ME, Ye YC, Chen SR, *et al.* Use of all-*trans* retinoic acid in the treatment of acute promyelocytic leukemia. Blood 1988; 72(2): 567-72.

[17]   Kastner P, Chambon P, Leid M. Role of nuclear retinoic acid receptors in the regulation of gene expression. Blomhoff R, editor. New York: Marcel Dekker; 1994.

[18]   Mangelsdorf DJ, Umesono K, Evans RM. The retinoid receptors. Sporn MB, Roberts, A.B., Goodman, D.S., editor. New York: Raven Press; 1994.

[19]   de The H, Chomienne C, Lanotte M, Degos L, Dejean A. The t(15;17) translocation of acute promyelocytic leukaemia fuses the retinoic acid receptor alpha gene to a novel transcribed locus. Nature 1990; 347(6293): 558-61.

[20]   de The H, Lavau C, Marchio A, *et al.* The PML-RAR alpha fusion mRNA generated by the t(15;17) translocation in acute promyelocytic leukemia encodes a functionally altered RAR. Cell 1991; 66(4): 675-84.

[21]   Lane MA, Bailey SJ. Role of retinoid signalling in the adult brain. Prog Neurobiol 2005; 75(4): 275-93.

[22]   Barnard JH, Collings JC, Whiting A, Przyborski SA, Marder TB. Synthetic Retinoids: Structure-Activity Relationships. Chemistry 2009.

[23]   Kawaguchi R, Yu J, Honda J, *et al.* A membrane receptor for retinol binding protein mediates cellular uptake of vitamin A. Science 2007; 315(5813): 820-5.

[24]   Gumireddy K, Sutton LN, Phillips PC, Reddy CD. All-*trans*-retinoic acid-induced apoptosis in human medulloblastoma: activation of caspase-3/poly(ADP-ribose) polymerase 1 pathway. Clin Cancer Res 2003; 9(11): 4052-9.

[25]   Heyman RA, Mangelsdorf DJ, Dyck JA, *et al.* 9-*cis* retinoic acid is a high affinity ligand for the retinoid X receptor. Cell 1992; 68(2): 397-406.

[26]   Levin AA, Sturzenbecker LJ, Kazmer S, *et al.* 9-*cis* retinoic acid stereoisomer binds and activates the nuclear receptor RXR alpha. Nature 1992; 355(6358): 359-61.

[27]   Soprano DR, Qin P, Soprano KJ. Retinoic acid receptors and cancers. Annu Rev Nutr 2004; 24: 201-21.

[28]   Idres N, Marill J, Flexor MA, Chabot GG. Activation of retinoic acid receptor-dependent transcription by all-*trans*-retinoic acid metabolites and isomers. J Biol Chem 2002; 277(35): 31491-8.

[29]   Tsukada M, Schroder M, Roos TC, *et al.* 13-*cis* retinoic acid exerts its specific activity on human sebocytes through selective intracellular isomerization to all-*trans* retinoic acid and binding to retinoid acid receptors. J Invest Dermatol 2000; 115(2): 321-7.

[30]   Shaw N, Elholm M, Noy N. Retinoic acid is a high affinity selective ligand for the peroxisome proliferator-activated receptor beta/delta. J Biol Chem 2003; 278(43): 41589-92.

[31]   Laudet V, Gronemeyer H. The Nuclear Receptor Facts. London: Academic Press; 2002.

[32]   Schug TT, Berry DC, Shaw NS, Travis SN, Noy N. Opposing effects of retinoic acid on cell growth result from alternate activation of two different nuclear receptors. Cell 2007; 129(4): 723-33.

[33]   Schug TT, Berry DC, Toshkov IA, *et al.* Overcoming retinoic acid-resistance of mammary carcinomas by diverting retinoic acid from PPARbeta/delta to RAR. Proc Natl Acad Sci U S A 2008; 105(21): 7546-51.

[34]   Mantymaa P, Guttorm T, Siitonen T, *et al.* Cellular redox state and its relationship to the inhibition of clonal cell growth and the induction of apoptosis during all-*trans* retinoic acid exposure in acute myeloblastic leukemia cells. Haematologica 2000; 85(3): 238-45.

[35]   Li JJ, Dong Z, Dawson MI, Colburn NH. Inhibition of tumor promoter-induced transformation by retinoids that transrepress AP-1 without transactivating retinoic acid response element. Cancer Res 1996; 56(3): 483-9.

[36]   Salbert G, Fanjul A, Piedrafita FJ, *et al.* Retinoic acid receptors and retinoid X receptor-alpha down-regulate the transforming growth factor-beta 1 promoter by antagonizing AP-1 activity. Mol Endocrinol 1993; 7(10): 1347-56.

[37]   Lovat PE, Irving H, Malcolm AJ, Pearson AD, Redfern CP. 9-*cis* retinoic acid--a better retinoid for the modulation of differentiation, proliferation and gene expression in human neuroblastoma. J Neurooncol 1997; 31(1-2): 85-91.

[38]   Lovat PE, Irving H, Annicchiarico-Petruzzelli M, *et al.* Retinoids in neuroblastoma therapy: distinct biological properties of 9-*cis*-and all-*trans*-retinoic acid. Eur J Cancer 1997; 33(12): 2075-80.

[39]   Ponthan F, Borgstrom P, Hassan M, *et al.* The vitamin A analogues: 13-*cis* retinoic acid, 9-*cis* retinoic acid, and Ro 13-6307 inhibit neuroblastoma tumour growth *in vivo*. Med Pediatr Oncol 2001; 36(1): 127-31.

[40]   Hansen NJ, Wylie RC, Phipps SM, *et al.* The low-toxicity 9-*cis* UAB30 novel retinoid down-regulates the DNA methyltransferases and has anti-telomerase activity in human breast cancer cells. Int J Oncol 2007; 30(3): 641-50.

[41]   Armstrong JL, Ruiz M, Boddy AV, *et al.* Increasing the intracellular availability of all-*trans* retinoic acid in neuroblastoma cells. Br J Cancer 2005; 92(4): 696-704.

[42]   Van Heusden J, Van Ginckel R, Bruwiere H, *et al.* Inhibition of all-*trans*-retinoic acid metabolism by R116010 induces antitumour activity. Br J Cancer 2002; 86(4): 605-11.

[43]   Danilenko M, Wang X, Studzinski GP. Carnosic acid and promotion of monocytic differentiation of HL60-G cells initiated by other agents. J Natl Cancer Inst 2001; 93(16): 1224-33.

[44]   Passeron T, Valencia JC, Namiki T, *et al.* Upregulation of SOX9 inhibits the growth of human and mouse melanomas and restores their sensitivity to retinoic acid. J Clin Invest 2009; 119(4): 954-63.

[45]   Seifried HE, Anderson DE, Fisher EI, Milner JA. A review of the interaction among dietary antioxidants and reactive oxygen species. J Nutr Biochem 2007; 18(9): 567-79.

[46]   Finkel T, Holbrook NJ. Oxidants, oxidative stress and the biology of ageing. Nature 2000; 408(6809): 239-47.

[47]   Park C, Jin CY, Kwon HJ, *et al.* Induction of apoptosis by esculetin in human leukemia U937 cells: Roles of Bcl-2 and extracellular-regulated kinase signaling. Toxicol *In vitro* 2009.

[48]   Witcher M, Ross DT, Rousseau C, Deluca L, Miller WH, Jr. Synergy between all-*trans* retinoic acid and tumor necrosis factor pathways in acute leukemia cells. Blood 2003; 102(1): 237-45.

[49]   Kiningham KK, Cardozo ZA, Cook C, *et al.* All-*trans*-retinoic acid induces manganese superoxide dismutase in human neuroblastoma through NF-kappaB. Free Radic Biol Med 2008; 44(8): 1610-6.

[50]   Feng Z, Porter AG. NF-kappaB/Rel proteins are required for neuronal differentiation of SH-SY5Y neuroblastoma cells. J Biol Chem 1999; 274(43): 30341-4.

[51]   Yoshida Y, Maruyama M, Fujita T, *et al.* Reactive oxygen intermediates stimulate interleukin-6 production in human bronchial epithelial cells. Am J Physiol 1999; 276(6 Pt 1): L900-8.

[52]   Balkwill F, Mantovani A. Inflammation and cancer: back to Virchow? Lancet 2001; 357(9255): 539-45.

[53]   Mueller MM, Fusenig NE. Friends or foes-bipolar effects of the tumour stroma in cancer. Nat Rev Cancer 2004; 4(11): 839-49.

[54]   Hussain SP, Harris CC. Inflammation and cancer: an ancient link with novel potentials. Int J Cancer 2007; 121(11): 2373-80.

[55]   Gelain DP, Moreira JC. Evidence of increased reactive species formation by retinol, but not retinoic acid, in PC12 cells. Toxicol *In vitro* 2008; 22(3): 553-8.

[56]   Delia D, Aiello A, Lombardi L, *et al.* N-(4-hydroxyphenyl)retinamide induces apoptosis of malignant hemopoietic cell lines including those unresponsive to retinoic acid. Cancer Res 1993; 53(24): 6036-41.

[57]   Oridate N, Suzuki S, Higuchi M, *et al.* Involvement of reactive oxygen species in N-(4-hydroxyphenyl)retinamide-induced apoptosis in cervical carcinoma cells. J Natl Cancer Inst 1997; 89(16): 1191-8.

[58]   Bu P, Wan YJ. Fenretinide-induced apoptosis of Huh-7 hepatocellular carcinoma is retinoic acid receptor beta dependent. BMC Cancer 2007; 7: 236.

[59]   Tsatmali M, Walcott EC, Makarenkova H, Crossin KL. Reactive oxygen species modulate the differentiation of neurons in clonal cortical cultures. Mol Cell Neurosci 2006; 33(4): 345-57.

[60]   Reddy NM, Kleeberger SR, Bream JH, *et al.* Genetic disruption of the Nrf2 compromises cell-cycle progression by impairing GSH-induced redox signaling. Oncogene 2008.

[61]   Castaigne S, Chomienne C, Daniel MT, *et al.* All-*trans* retinoic acid as a differentiation therapy for acute promyelocytic leukemia. I. Clinical results. Blood 1990; 76(9): 1704-9.

[62]   Zhang JW, Wang JY, Chen SJ, Chen Z. Mechanisms of all-*trans* retinoic acid-induced differentiation of acute promyelocytic leukemia cells. J Biosci 2000; 25(3): 275-84.

[63]   Benoit G, Altucci L, Flexor M, *et al.* RAR-independent RXR signaling induces t(15;17) leukemia cell maturation. Embo J 1999; 18(24): 7011-8.

[64]   Konopka R, Kubala L, Lojek A, Pachernik J. Alternation of retinoic acid induced neural differentiation of P19 embryonal carcinoma cells by reduction of reactive oxygen species intracellular production. Neuro Endocrinol Lett 2008; 29(5): 770-4.

[65]   Nefedova Y, Fishman M, Sherman S, *et al.* Mechanism of all-*trans* retinoic acid effect on tumor-associated myeloid-derived suppressor cells. Cancer Res 2007; 67(22): 11021-8.

[66]   Kusmartsev S, Nefedova Y, Yoder D, Gabrilovich DI. Antigen-specific inhibition of CD8+ T cell response by immature myeloid cells in cancer is mediated by reactive oxygen species. J Immunol 2004; 172(2): 989-99.

[67]   Kusmartsev S, Gabrilovich DI. Inhibition of myeloid cell differentiation in cancer: the role of reactive oxygen species. J Leukoc Biol 2003; 74(2): 186-96.

[68]   Dickinson DA, Forman HJ. Glutathione in defense and signaling: lessons from a small thiol. Ann N Y Acad Sci 2002; 973: 488-504.

[69]   Chomienne C, Ballerini P, Balitrand N, *et al.* All-*trans* retinoic acid in acute promyelocytic leukemias. II. *In vitro* studies: structure-function relationship. Blood 1990; 76(9): 1710-7.

[70]   Yen A, Albright KL. Evidence for cell cycle phase-specific initiation of a program of HL-60 cell myeloid differentiation mediated by inducer uptake. Cancer Res 1984; 44(6): 2511-5.

[71]   Crow JP. Dichlorodihydrofluorescein and dihydrorhodamine 123 are sensitive indicators of peroxynitrite *in vitro*: implications for intracellular measurement of reactive nitrogen and oxygen species. Nitric Oxide 1997; 1(2): 145-57.

[72]   Matthay KK, Villablanca JG, Seeger RC, *et al.* Treatment of high-risk neuroblastoma with intensive chemotherapy, radiotherapy, autologous bone marrow transplantation, and 13-*cis*-retinoic acid. Children's Cancer Group. N Engl J Med 1999; 341(16): 1165-73.

[73]   Cuende J, Moreno S, Bolanos JP, Almeida A. Retinoic acid downregulates Rae1 leading to APC(Cdh1) activation and neuroblastoma SH-SY5Y differentiation. Oncogene 2008; 27(23): 3339-44.

[74]   Wainwright LJ, Lasorella A, Iavarone A. Distinct mechanisms of cell cycle arrest control the decision between differentiation and senescence in human neuroblastoma cells. Proc Natl Acad Sci U S A 2001; 98(16): 9396-400.

[75]   Liu M, Iavarone A, Freedman LP. Transcriptional activation of the human p21(WAF1/CIP1) gene by retinoic acid receptor. Correlation with retinoid induction of U937 cell differentiation. J Biol Chem 1996; 271(49): 31723-8.

[76]   Catalano S, Giordano C, Rizza P, *et al.* Evidence that leptin through STAT and CREB signaling enhances cyclin D1 expression and promotes human endometrial cancer proliferation. J Cell Physiol 2009; 218(3): 490-500.

[77]   Liao DJ, Thakur A, Wu J, Biliran H, Sarkar FH. Perspectives on c-Myc, Cyclin D1, and their interaction in cancer formation, progression, and response to chemotherapy. Crit Rev Oncog 2007; 13(2): 93-158.

[78]   Raelson JV, Nervi C, Rosenauer A, *et al.* The PML/RAR alpha oncoprotein is a direct molecular target of retinoic acid in acute promyelocytic leukemia cells. Blood 1996; 88(8): 2826-32.

[79]   Yoshida H, Kitamura K, Tanaka K, *et al.* Accelerated degradation of PML-retinoic acid receptor alpha (PML-RARA) oncoprotein by all-*trans*-retinoic acid in acute promyelocytic leukemia: possible role of the proteasome pathway. Cancer Res 1996; 56(13): 2945-8.

[80]   Nervi C, Ferrara FF, Fanelli M, *et al.* Caspases mediate retinoic acid-induced degradation of the acute promyelocytic leukemia PML/RARalpha fusion protein. Blood 1998; 92(7): 2244-51.

[81]   Zhu J, Gianni M, Kopf E, *et al.* Retinoic acid induces proteasome-dependent degradation of retinoic acid receptor alpha (RARalpha) and oncogenic RARalpha fusion proteins. Proc Natl Acad Sci U S A 1999; 96(26): 14807-12.

[82]   Privalle CT, Fridovich I. Induction of superoxide dismutase in Escherichia coli by heat shock. Proc Natl Acad Sci U S A 1987; 84(9): 2723-6.

[83]   Culotta VC, Yang M, O'Halloran TV. Activation of superoxide dismutases: putting the metal to the pedal. Biochim Biophys Acta 2006; 1763(7): 747-58.

[84]   Erlejman AG, Oteiza PI. The oxidant defense system in human neuroblastoma IMR-32 cells prediferentiation and postdifferentiation to neuronal phenotypes. Neurochem Res 2002; 27(11): 1499-506.

[85]   Hansberg W, de Groot H, Sies H. Reactive oxygen species associated with cell differentiation in Neurospora crassa. Free Radic Biol Med 1993; 14(3): 287-93.

[86]   Oberley LW, Ridnour LA, Sierra-Rivera E, Oberley TD, Guernsey DL. Superoxide dismutase activities of differentiating clones from an immortal cell line. J Cell Physiol 1989; 138(1): 50-60.

[87]   Canon E, Cosgaya JM, Scsucova S, Aranda A. Rapid effects of retinoic acid on CREB and ERK phosphorylation in neuronal cells. Mol Biol Cell 2004; 15(12): 5583-92.

[88]   Aggarwal S, Kim SW, Cheon K, *et al.* Nonclassical action of retinoic acid on the activation of the cAMP response element-binding protein in normal human bronchial epithelial cells. Mol Biol Cell 2006; 17(2): 566-75.

[89]   Washio A, Kitamura C, Jimi E, Terashita M, Nishihara T. Mechanisms involved in suppression of NGF-induced neuronal differentiation of PC12 cells by hyaluronic acid. Exp Cell Res 2009; 315(17): 3036-43.

[90]   McManus MF, Chen LC, Vallejo I, Vallejo M. Astroglial differentiation of cortical precursor cells triggered by activation of the cAMP-dependent signaling pathway. J Neurosci 1999; 19(20): 9004-15.

[91]   Atencia R, Garcia-Sanz M, Unda F, Arechaga J. Apoptosis during retinoic acid-induced differentiation of F9 embryonal carcinoma cells. Exp Cell Res 1994; 214(2): 663-7.

[92]   Clifford J, Chiba H, Sobieszczuk D, Metzger D, Chambon P. RXRalpha-null F9 embryonal carcinoma cells are resistant to the differentiation, anti-proliferative and apoptotic effects of retinoids. Embo J 1996; 15(16): 4142-55.

[93]   Boylan JF, Lohnes D, Taneja R, Chambon P, Gudas LJ. Loss of retinoic acid receptor gamma function in F9 cells by gene disruption results in aberrant Hoxa-1 expression and differentiation upon retinoic acid treatment. Proc Natl Acad Sci U S A 1993; 90(20): 9601-5.

[94]   Boylan JF, Lufkin T, Achkar CC, *et al.* Targeted disruption of retinoic acid receptor alpha (RAR alpha) and RAR gamma results in receptor-specific alterations in retinoic acid-mediated differentiation and retinoic acid metabolism. Mol Cell Biol 1995; 15(2): 843-51.

[95]   Chiba H, Clifford J, Metzger D, Chambon P. Distinct retinoid X receptor-retinoic acid receptor heterodimers are differentially involved in the control of expression of retinoid target genes in F9 embryonal carcinoma cells. Mol Cell Biol 1997; 17(6): 3013-20.

[96]   Chiba H, Clifford J, Metzger D, Chambon P. Specific and redundant functions of retinoid X Receptor/Retinoic acid receptor heterodimers in differentiation, proliferation, and apoptosis of F9 embryonal carcinoma cells. J Cell Biol 1997; 139(3): 735-47.

[97]   Sheikh MS, Shao ZM, Li XS, *et al.* N-(4-hydroxyphenyl)retinamide (4-HPR)-mediated biological actions involve retinoid receptor-independent pathways in human breast carcinoma. Carcinogenesis 1995; 16(10): 2477-86.

[98]   Oridate N, Lotan D, Xu XC, Hong WK, Lotan R. Differential induction of apoptosis by all-*trans*-retinoic acid and N-(4-hydroxyphenyl)retinamide in human head and neck squamous cell carcinoma cell lines. Clin Cancer Res 1996; 2(5): 855-63.

[99]   Clifford JL, Menter DG, Wang M, Lotan R, Lippman SM. Retinoid receptor-dependent and-independent effects of N-(4-hydroxyphenyl)retinamide in F9 embryonal carcinoma cells. Cancer Res 1999; 59(1): 14-8.

[100] Delia D, Aiello A, Formelli F, *et al.* Regulation of apoptosis induced by the retinoid N-(4-hydroxyphenyl) retinamide and effect of deregulated bcl-2. Blood 1995; 85(2): 359-67.

[101] Myhre O, Andersen JM, Aarnes H, Fonnum F. Evaluation of the probes 2',7'-dichlorofluorescin diacetate, luminol, and lucigenin as indicators of reactive species formation. Biochem Pharmacol 2003; 65(10): 1575-82.

[102] Tew KD. Glutathione-associated enzymes in anticancer drug resistance. Cancer Res 1994; 54(16): 4313-20.

[103] O'Dwyer PJ, Hamilton TC, Yao KS, Tew KD, Ozols RF. Modulation of glutathione and related enzymes in reversal of resistance to anticancer drugs. Hematol Oncol Clin North Am 1995; 9(2): 383-96.

[104] Wang ZG, Delva L, Gaboli M, *et al.* Role of PML in cell growth and the retinoic acid pathway. Science 1998; 279(5356): 1547-51.

[105] Wang ZG, Ruggero D, Ronchetti S, *et al.* PML is essential for multiple apoptotic pathways. Nat Genet 1998; 20(3): 266-72.

[106] Kast RE. Potential for all-*trans* retinoic acid (tretinoin) to enhance interferon-alpha treatment response in chronic myelogenous leukemia, melanoma, myeloma and renal cell carcinoma. Cancer Biol Ther 2008; 7(10): 1515-9.

[107] Garbe C, Eigentler TK. Diagnosis and treatment of cutaneous melanoma: state of the art 2006. Melanoma Res 2007; 17(2): 117-27.

[108] Spanjaard RA, Lee PJ, Sarkar S, Goedegebuure PS, Eberlein TJ. Clone 10d/BM28 (CDCL1), an early S-phase protein, is an important growth regulator of melanoma. Cancer Res 1997; 57(22): 5122-8.

[109] Zhao X, Demary K, Wong L, *et al.* Retinoic acid receptor-independent mechanism of apoptosis of melanoma cells by the retinoid CD437 (AHPN). Cell Death Differ 2001; 8(9): 878-86.

[110] Wang H, Maurer BJ, Liu YY, *et al.* N-(4-Hydroxyphenyl)retinamide increases dihydroceramide and synergizes with dimethylsphingosine to enhance cancer cell killing. Mol Cancer Ther 2008; 7(9): 2967-76.

[111] Park EY, Dillard A, Williams EA, *et al.* Retinol inhibits the growth of all-*trans*-retinoic acid-sensitive and all-*trans*-retinoic acid-resistant colon cancer cells through a retinoic acid receptor-independent mechanism. Cancer Res 2005; 65(21): 9923-33.

[112] Basu TK, Chan UM, Fields AL, McPherson TA. Retinol and postoperative colorectal cancer patients. Br J Cancer 1985; 51(1): 61-5.

[113] Park EY, Wilder ET, Lane MA. Retinol inhibits the invasion of retinoic acid-resistant colon cancer cells *in vitro* and decreases matrix metalloproteinase mRNA, protein, and activity levels. Nutr Cancer 2007; 57(1): 66-77.

CHAPTER 6

Epigenetics as a Mechanism for Dietary Fatty Acids to Affect Hematopoietic Stem/Progenitor Cells And Leukemia - Royal Jelly for the Blood

Vincent E. Sollars[*]

Nutrition and Cancer Center, Department of Biochemistry and Microbiology, Joan C. Edwards School of Medicine, Marshall University, Huntington, WV, 25705, USA

Abstract: In this chapter, the impact of lipid molecules on hematopoiesis will be reviewed in a format friendly to those outside the field. The focus of the review is on how dietary fatty acids impact hematopoiesis through changes in differentiation. We begin with a discussion of general hematopoiesis including the concepts of stem and progenitor cells that drive hematopoiesis and the various cell types they produce. We then will discuss the principles of epigenetic gene regulation and differentiation pertinent to hematopoietic stem and progenitor cells. Once these principles have been introduced, we will examine how dietary lipids can impact hematopoietic differentiation. The relationship of epigenetics and dietary lipids to leukemic and preleukemic states will also be explored. We will conclude with a look at how WNT signaling can impact hematopoiesis through epigenetic gene regulation, dietary lipids, and differentiation.

Keywords: Cancer, Cyclooxygenase, Diet, Epigenetics, Fatty Acid, Fish, Fish Oil, Food, Hematological Cancer, Hematopoietic Stem Cells, Leukemia, Nutrition, Omega-3, Progenitor, Stem Cells, Wnt.

INTRODUCTION

The idea that environmental influences, such as diet, can produce changes in an organism is well established. That these same influences can elicit enduring effects that are capable of shaping offspring for several generations is a realization that holds vast potential and complication for human health. In this chapter, we will explore what is known about the ability of lipids in the diet to affect changes of this nature in the hematopoietic system.

The potential for human health that remains to be discovered in dietary influences is best illustrated in the honey bee [1]. The two diploid morphologies that exist in *Apis mellifera* can be produced from identical eggs by differential feeding of the larvae. Worker bees are produced from larvae fed a diet of nectar and pollen, while queen bees are produced when these larvae are fed large amounts of royal jelly. Nutritional differences during the development of these organisms not only result in different morphologies, but in different behavioral patterns and a 10 times longer lifespan for the queen. The nutritional induced differences were shown to be produced through DNA methylation by injecting larvae with a small interfering RNA targeting DNA methyltransferase 3 [2, 3]. Treated larvae produced a majority of queens in these experiments. These effects on the honey bee are very dramatic, more dramatic than what we will most likely see in nutritional effects on human health, yet they are illustrative of the potential that diet induced epigenetic change can have on an organism.

In this chapter, we will discuss the principles of hematopoietic stem and progenitor cells. What is known of the role of epigenetics in these processes will be presented, as well as the effects dietary lipids have on these processes.

---
*Address Correspondence to Vincent E. Sollars:** Nutrition and Cancer Center, Department of Biochemistry and Microbiology, Joan C. Edwards School of Medicine, Marshall University, Byrd Biotechnology Science Center, Room 336N, 1700 Third Avenue, Huntington WV, 25755, USA; E-mail: sollars@marshall.edu

HEMATOPOIETIC STEM AND PROGENITOR CELLS

Stem cells are the cells responsible for production of new tissues during development or replacement of damaged tissue, such as wound closing in adults. Hematopoietic stem cells (HSCs) are responsible for the production of the diverse cell types present in the blood and lymph, but only comprise about 0.01% of the cells present in the bone marrow [4]. HSCs were first described in 1961 by Till and MCCulloch [5]. Stem cells have two characteristics that define them. First, they are immortal in that there is no limit to the number of times they can undergo mitosis. Normal cells have a defined lifespan measured in cellular divisions before they enter a quiescent state known as senescence. Normal cells are only capable of 50-75 cellular divisions before undergoing senescence (the Hayflick limit [6]), whereas stem cells do not have this restriction. During hematopoiesis (Fig. 1), this is the first characteristic that is diminished during the differentiation process from long-term hematopoietic stem cells (LT-HSC) to short-term hematopoietic stem cells (ST-HSC), which is eventually lost in becoming the multipotential progenitor cell. Second, stem cells are pluripotent with the capacity to mature into multiple cell types. In hematopoiesis, stem cells are capable of producing the various myeloid and lymphoid lineages such as B-cells, T-cells, neutrophils, *etc.* [7]. Pluripotency is gradually lost as hematopoietic stem cells (HSCs) differentiate to the various classes of progenitor cells and finally into their terminally differentiated counterparts (Fig. 1). Progenitors gradually decrease their capacity to produce diverse cell types, until they become committed progenitors capable of generating a single cell type. During the differentiation process of hematopoiesis several cellular characteristics change that are pertinent to the process of generating cancers of the blood, leukemogenesis. We have already discussed the loss of immortality, a characteristic of cancerous cells [8], in going from a stem cell state to a progenitor. Cellular proliferation rates also change during hematopoiesis. Hematopoietic differentiation is based upon the need to replace about five hundred billion blood cells in the human body each day [9]. The HSC does not generate the required 5×10^{11} cells directly on a daily basis, but instead generates highly prolific progenitor cells that produce the major hematopoietic cell types (Fig. 1). These progenitor cells serve the function of cellular amplification between the largely quiescent HSC and the non-dividing mature cell.

Cancer stem cells share many characteristics with normal stem cells. A minor fraction of the tumor contains these cells that are responsible for propagating the disease. They are thought to be the primary agent for recurrence of the disease after remission. Cancer stem cells, like normal stem cells, are largely quiescent and are refractory to cancer therapies that generally target the rapidly dividing nature of cancer cells. In leukemias, such as AML, leukemia stem cells have been found to have long-term and short-term repopulating abilities when transferred to new hosts, much like normal HSCs [10-12]. It is still unknown, whether the leukemia stem cell originates from an HSC or from a progenitor cell that reacquires stem cell characteristics. The most recent evidence suggests that the progenitor cell is the cell of origin of the leukemic stem cell. Indeed, the granulocyte monocyte progenitor (Fig. 1) has been proposed as a candidate leukemic stem cell for blast-crisis chronic myelogenous leukemia [13] and early progenitors have been postulated as the leukemic stem cell in acute lymphoid leukemia [14]. In addition to studies in humans, studies in the mouse model have provided valuable evidence for progenitor cells as the origin of leukemic stem cells [15-18]. Andrew Feinberg, the discoverer of the connection between epigenetics and cancer, has postulated that progenitor cell dynamics and epigenetic gene regulation are predominant factors in leukemogenesis [19]. Indeed, the realization that stem cells are largely defined by their epigenetic state makes the progenitor cell as the cell of origin for leukemia a likely hypothesis.

EPIGENETICS AND HEMATOPOIETIC STEM CELLS

It has become apparent that one of the key factors that maintains stem cells in their state is a particular epigenetic configuration [20-23]. Epigenetics is defined as mitotically heritable modifications of DNA or chromatin that do not alter the primary nucleotide sequence. The type of regulatory networks included in epigenetics are histone post-translational modifications and histone variants, as well as cytosine methylation of DNA. Over the last few years, there have been several studies attempting to decode the epigenetic regulatory signals involved in maintaining the stem cell state. Before discussing the epigenetics of stem cells we will review the primary mechanisms of epigenetic gene regulation.

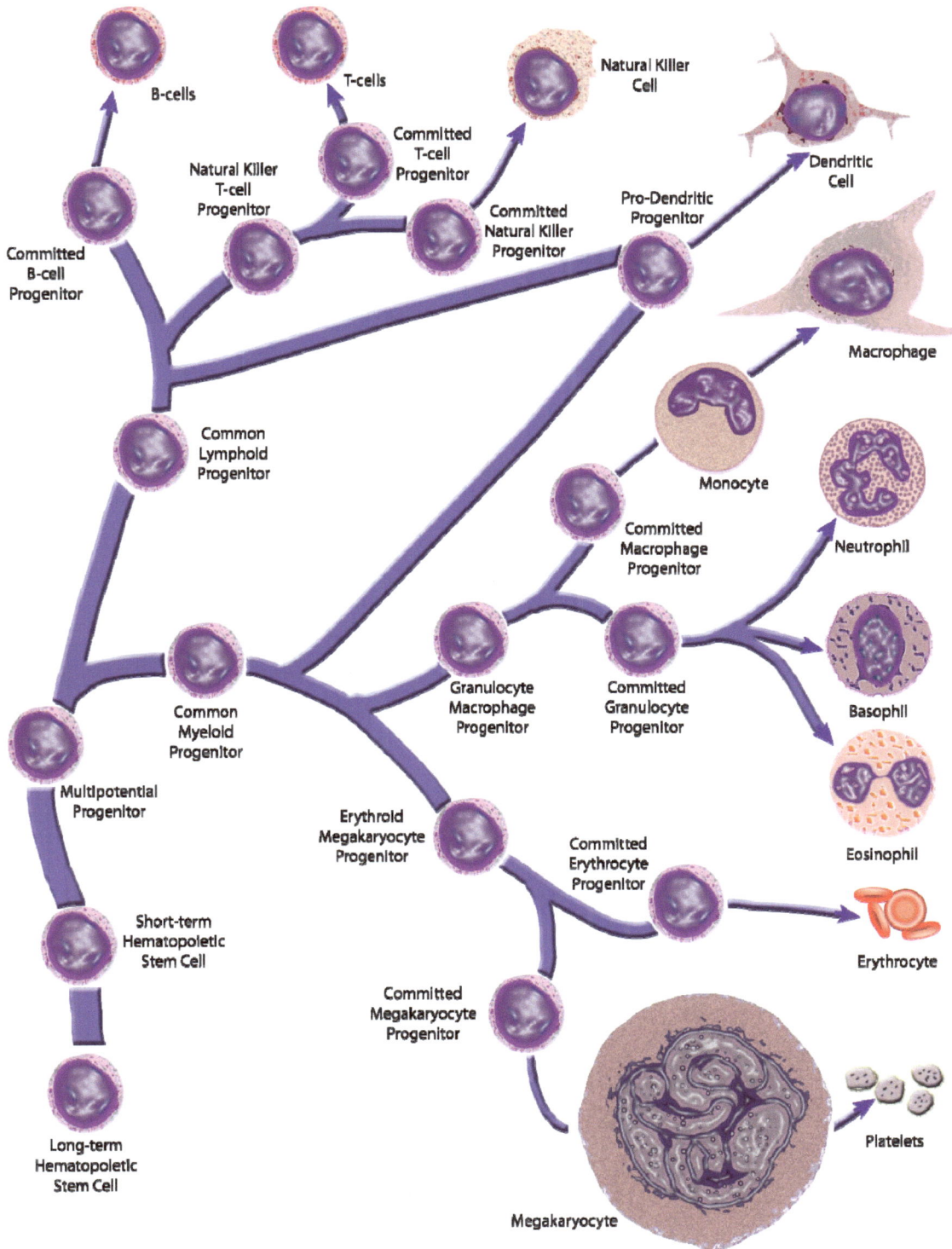

Figure 1: Hematopoietic stem and progenitor cell maturation. The maturation process of stem and progenitor cells in hematopoietic tissue is shown. Maturation proceeds from the hematopoietic stem cell to the multipotential progenitor cell. This first progenitor cell in the lineage produces the two progenitors capable of generating the lymphoid or myeloid arms of the immune system, the common myeloid progenitor and the common lymphoid progenitor. Each of these progenitors progressively loses cell fate options until they finally become committed progenitors capable of only producing a single cell type. The relative thickness of the lines illustrates the developmental potential still present for the cell types.

Histones can undergo a variety of post-translational modifications including methylation, acetylation, phosphorylation, and ubiquitination that can interact with each other to determine the effect on chromatin structure [24-26]. Allis has formulated a "histone code" hypothesis that suggests that the timing, type, placement, and sequence of histone posttranslational modifications comprises a code for protein recruitment, substrate specificity and chromatin remodeling in service of transcriptional control [27]. The most well characterized effect is that of histone acetylation, which has the effect of opening chromatin structure to increase accessibility of genes to trans-acting factors such as transcription factors and RNA polymerase. Histone acetylases add acetyl groups to histones, while histone deacetylases remove them. In addition to modification of the four conserved histone proteins (H2A, H2B, H3, and H4), several other variants exist for H2A (H2A.X, H2A.Z, H2A-Bbd, and MacroH2A) and H3 (H3.1, H3.2, H3.3, and CenpA). Unlike normal histones, these variants are assembled into chromatin independently of DNA replication. They have diverse roles ranging from X-chromosome inactivation [28, 29] and protection of euchromatin [30]. There is also evidence that histone variants are involved in regulating embryonic stem cell differentiation and possibly pluripotency [31].

Methylation of cytosines in DNA occurs at the 5 position carbon in the ribose ring by the activity of DNA methyltransferases [32]. This has two primary mechanisms of affecting the expression of genes. First, the methyl group acts to sterically inhibit interaction of trans-acting factors with the DNA in that region. This often results in repressing expression of genes, *e.g.* when these occur in the promoter regions of genes to inhibit the interaction of RNA polymerase and transcription factors. However, DNA methylation can also result in activation of genes if these methylation events occur in the binding sites of transcriptional repressors, such as in the *Il8* gene in breast cancer [33]. The second mechanism by which cytosine methylation affects DNA is through the binding of proteins of the methyl-CpG-binding domain proteins (MBDs) and methyl-CpG binding protein (MeCP) families that recruit transcription-repressing complexes affecting histone modification such as histone deacetylases [34] and histone methylases [35, 36].

The connection between epigenetic gene regulation and stem cells is the pervasive involvement of epigenetic gene regulation during the process of differentiation, which stem cells are also intimately connected with as the mother cell of the cells belonging to their respective lineages. The methylation and acetylation states of DNA can induce structural changes in chromatin that activate gene expression during differentiation [37-39]. An early insight into the transcriptional profile of HSCs was provided by the Weissman laboratory with gene expression profiling of murine hematopoietic stem and progenitor cells purified by fluorescence activated cell sorting [40]. These studies found that HSCs contained almost half of the differentially expressed genes and the respective progenitor cells having about ten percent on average of the differentially expressed genes. These results indicated that though HSCs appear quiescent they are quite active as far as control of transcription. Evidence indicates that the transcriptional control activity hinted at in these studies is of an epigenetic nature. Stem cells rely on Polycomb group proteins, which repress gene expression though epigenetic mechanisms, to reversibly repress genes encoding transcription factors required for differentiation [41, 42]. Bmi-1, a polycomb protein, critically regulates self-renewal of different adult stem cell populations through inhibition of p16 expression and its alternative reading frame [43-45].

One key aspect of stem cell transcriptional control that has recently come to light is the idea that loci important to cell fate decisions are placed in a "poised" state of transcriptional activation through epigenetic gene regulation. This poised state is mediated by having histones bivalently marked (having both repressive and activating marks) in the genes of interest [46, 47]. Studies in mouse embryonic stem cells found that several important silent developmental genes such as *Irx3, Nkx2.2, Pax3* and *Sox1* were found in fractions enriched for the repressive H3K27me3 and activating H3K4me3/H3K9ac3 histone modifications [48]. This work was supported by later investigations targeting the lineage control genes *POU, Pax, Sox*, and *Hox* in embryonic stem cells [49]. In these studies, not only did they find these genes to be bivalently marked, but these patterns were erased upon differentiation into neuronal progenitor cells. Neuronal specific genes lost the H3K27me3 repressive mark, but retained the H3K4me3 active mark. Silent pluripotent genes exhibited the converse pattern. This pattern of poised transcription mediated through bivalent histone modifications is also seen in human T cell development [50].

The homeobox gene family of transcription factors (or Hox gene family in mammalian systems) is responsible for delineating cell fates. These are transcription factors expressed during differentiation that elicit changes in gene expression necessary for commitment of a cell to a particular cell fate, inducing morphological and physiological transformations of the cell. The non-human mammalian counterparts to the 39 human homeobox class I genes are best known for their roles in axial patterning during development [51]. The trithorax group (Trx-G) and polycomb group (Pc-G) genes were initially characterized in *Drosophila* and yeast as regulators of transcription through chromatin remodeling, an epigenetic mechanism. The Trx-G genes maintain stable transcription of genes, while the Pc-G genes are responsible for gene silencing. These two gene families act antagonistically to control the expression of the homeobox transcription factor gene family by providing cellular memory of cell fate decisions. Since the homeobox genes are under control of the Trx-G and Pc-G genes, mutations in these two gene families result in loss of regulated expression of the homeobox genes and aberrations in cell lineage decisions.

Identification of factors that are involved in making differentiation choices, *i.e.* cellular commitment, is extremely important in our treatment of leukemia. The relationship between lineage commitment and leukemia is best understood through the study of the homeobox (Hox) class of genes. In 1988, Hox genes were linked to murine leukemic transformation when the WEHI-3B leukemic cell line was found to contain proviral integrations resulting in transcriptional activation of Hoxb8 and Interleukin 3 (Il3) [52]. Later, direct evidence for Hox involvement in leukemic transformation was reported when mice transplanted with bone marrow cells engineered to overexpress Hoxb8 and Il3 were shown to suffer from acute, aggressive, polyclonal leukemia [53]. Other Hox genes have also been implicated in leukemia, including Tlx1, Hoxa9, Hoxa10, and Hoxb3 [54-57]. Conservation of Hox-induced leukemic transformation between mice and humans is indicated by the recurrent reciprocal translocation t(7;11), predominantly associated with acute myelogenous leukemia (AML). This translocation results in a fusion of a subdomain of NUP38, a member of the GLFG nucleoporin family, with HOXA9 [58]. Evidence has continued to accumulate implicating other Hox genes in leukemia, including *myeloid ecotropic integration site 1* (*Meis1*) [56, 59]. This gene has been found to be inactivated in acute myelogenous leukemia (AML) by hypermethylation [60] and its cofactors in leukemic transformation, HoxA7 and HoxA9, have been found to be expressed in HSCs [40].

Myelodysplastic syndrome (MDS), myeloproliferative disease (MPD), and AML are related hematopoietic malignancies in that MDS and MPD often progress to AML. AML is characterized by loss of regulation of cell lineage decisions, resulting in the over-proliferation of immature myeloid cells. The impact of epigenetics in leukemia is seen in multiple significant examples. These epigenetic effects include increased methylation of the Pa promoter of *Abl* seen in advanced phases of chronic myelogenous leukemia (CML) [61, 62], in addition to methylation of *Bcr* in lymphoid blast crisis [63]. Hypermethylation of *p15*, an inhibitor of cyclin-dependent kinase 4 (CDK4) and CDK6, is also associated with CML transformation [64]. The importance of *p15* is seen in disease progression from MDS to AML, where *p15* is targeted for hypermethylation in 78% of samples at the time of leukemic transformation [65]. Also, increased expression levels of the DNA methyltransferase (DNMT) genes *DNMT1*, *DNMT3A*, and *DNMT3B* correlate with blast phase CML [66]. Another factor related to cytosine methylation that is pertinent to cancer is that DNA methylation of cytosines at CpG sites increases the rate of mutations of methylated cytosines by an order of magnitude [67]. Epigenetics may be a significantly more important mechanism in AML progression than in other cancers, because chromosomal instability does not seem to be predominant (57.6% *de novo* AML patients have normal cytogenetics) [68]. Hypermethylation as a mechanism of gene regulation is seen frequently in AML, and may be more frequent in young adults where AML is the most common form of leukemia [69].

LIPIDS AND HEMATOPOIETIC STEM/PROGENITOR CELLS

The effects of lipids and their metabolites on hematopoietic stem and progenitor cells have been inconclusive and often at conflict, most likely due to artifacts associated with cell culture. An example exemplifying this is the investigation of prostaglandin E_2 (PGE2). PGE2 has been the object of research for over 30 years to determine its role in regulating hematopoiesis. PGE2 is produced by the action of cyclooxygenase (COX)-1 or-2 on arachidonic acid to produce PGH2, that is further converted to PGE2 by prostaglandin synthases. Research on the effects of PGE2 on hematopoiesis has produced varying results on progenitor cells [70-75], mostly likely due to a combination of issues with the short half-life of PGE2 *in vivo*, the concentration used, and the length of exposure [76]. There is now strong *in vivo* evidence that PGE2 acts on HSCs to expand their numbers in mouse models [77-79]. Additionally, hematopoietic lineage regeneration is impaired in COX-2 deficient mice [80]. PGE2 has also been shown to have effects on hematopoietic progenitor cells. Micromolar concentrations of prostaglandin E2 effect human myeloid progenitor cell proliferation [81]. COX signaling and PGE2 have been shown to have roles in lymphoid progenitors in the zebrafish and mouse [82-84] and in myeloid progenitor cell maturation in humans and mice [81, 85-87].

Investigators interested in the effects of lipids on hematopoiesis have also investigated the precursor molecules of the prostaglandins, polyunsaturated fatty acids (Fig. **2**). The effects of polyunsaturated fatty acids, those containing more than one double bond in the carbon chain, are more diverse in that they are also metabolized to other eicosanoids such as leukotrienes, prostacyclin, resolvins, and thromboxanes, as well as incorporated into cell signaling molecules such as hedgehog and WNT [88]. The effects of the omega-3 (n-3) fatty acids α linolenic acid (ALA, 18:3), eicosapentaenoic acid (EPA, 20:5), and docosahexaenoic acid (DHA, 22:6), as well as the omega-6 (n-6) fatty acids linoleic acid (LNA, 18 carbons) and arachidonic acid (ARA, 20 carbons) have been of particular interest. N-3 and n-6 fatty acids from the diet are incorporated into cell membranes or processed. Processing occurs through elongation or β-oxidation followed by desaturation by Δ6 and Δ5 desaturases. Dietary linoleic acid is generally considered to be the major source of tissue arachidonic acid although meat fat can be a direct source of arachidonic acid [89]. N-3 fatty acids have greater affinity for the Δ5 and Δ6 desaturases than omega 6 fatty acids. Consequently, increasing dietary intake of n-3 fatty acids reduces the desaturation of linoleic acid and reduces the production of arachidonic acid [90]. All three major n-3 fatty acids directly inhibit the production of arachidonic acid from linoleic acid [90]. Both arachidonic acid and eicosapentaenoic acid can be cleaved from the cell membrane phospholipids stores by phospholipase A_2 and acted on by cyclooxygenases (either the constitutive COX1 or the inducible COX2) to produce prostaglandins. COX activity on arachidonic acid forms the 2-series prostaglandins that tend to be pro-proliferative and pro-inflammatory in most tissues [91]. However, COX activity on eicosapentaenoic acid forms the 3 series prostaglandins that tend to have anti-proliferative and anti-inflammatory properties [91]. Suppression of omega 6 derived eicosanoids has been proposed as a strategy for chemoprevention and as an adjunct for treatment of cancer [92-95].

Our investigations on the effects of changes in dietary n-3 and n-6 fatty acids in mice indicate that diet can influence the differentiation of progenitor cells of the myeloid variety [96, 97]. Our initial investigations were into later stage myeloid progenitors, those progenitors that have matured past the common myeloid progenitor (Fig. **1**). We found that dietary n-3 fatty acids produced more differentiated progenitors and less of them in the bone marrow of mice [96]. Our later experiments investigated the HSCs and earlier myeloid progenitor cells and found no change in the number of HSCs with n-3 *vs.* n-6 fatty acid rich diets, but we did find an increase in the frequency of the common myeloid progenitor with diets rich in n-3 fatty acids [97]. This suggests that diets rich in n-3 fatty acids produce delays in differentiation of the common myeloid progenitor, causing a reduction in the later stage progenitors of the myeloid lineages. Thus, diet can effect changes in the steady state level of differentiation in the mouse, but not necessarily differentiation potential or immortality of stem cells. It remains to be seen whether the dietary agents used in these studies are operating through an epigenetic mechanism. However, there is evidence for a connection between lipid metabolism and epigenetic gene regulation in that microarray analysis of honeybees fed royal jelly and RNAi silencing of DNA methyltransferase 3 in honeybees lead to changes in genes involved in lipid metabolism [2, 98].

LIPIDS AND THE WNT PATHWAY

The WNT pathway is prevalent during developmental and other signaling events in animal cells [99], including the maintenance of HSCs [100, 101]. The WNT signaling pathway is one of the four major pathways in hematopoietic stem/progenitor cell biology [102]. Two important connections between the WNT pathway and fatty acid metabolism have surfaced recently. First, WNT proteins have been found to undergo palmitoylation, the covalent attachment of fatty acids, on a conserved cysteine residue (C77 in the mouse Wnt3a) that is necessary for function [103]. Furthermore, these investigators found that palmitoylation was necessary to maintain HSC self-renewal in an *in vitro* model. Second, clinical evidence from colon cancer patients, in addition to cancer cell lines, suggests an association between WNT and PGE2 signalling [104-106]. This was supported by evidence in zebrafish, where it was found that PGE2 signaling stabilized β-catenin by phosphorylation [107]. Since WNT signaling also relies upon stabilized β-catenin, this is the likely candidate for interaction between these pathways. Interestingly, there is evidence from human cancer cell lines that COX-2 derived PGE2 activates β-catenin and n-3 fatty acids such as DPA and EPA inhibit this effect [108]. Thus, n-3 fatty acids may exert effects on the WNT pathway through this mechanism. If it is true that the WNT pathway is responsive to fatty acid levels and type in normal and abnormal human hematopoiesis, then there are potentially immense implications for blood and other cancers where the WNT pathway is an important pathway.

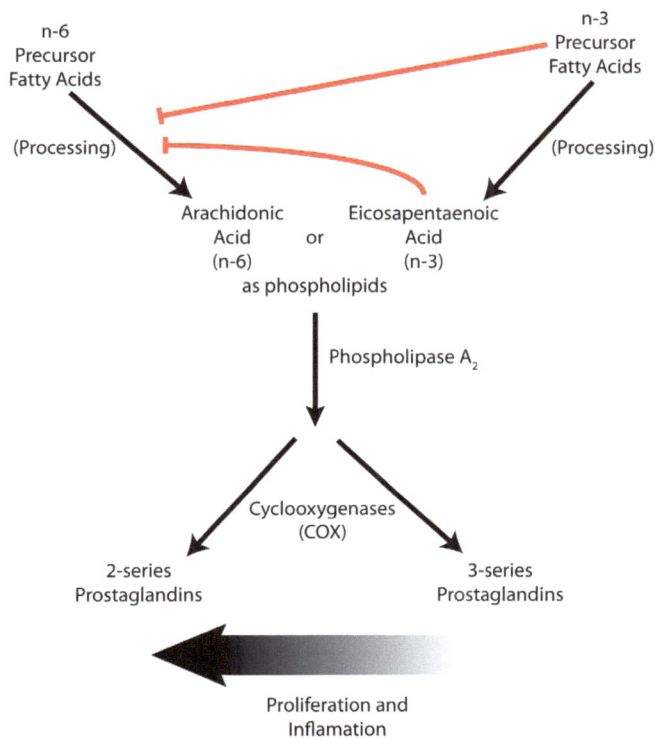

Figure 2: Omega fatty acids in prostaglandin formation. Precursor fatty acids are processed by elongation (addition of 2 carbons) or β-oxidation (removal of 2 carbons) to form 20 carbon chains that are then desaturated to form arachidonic or eicosa pentaenoic acid. The n-3 fatty acids will inhibit the production of arachidonic acid from the primary precursor, which is linoleic acid. Both fatty acid types are stored in phospholipid stores that can be released by the action of phospholipase A$_2$, and then acted upon by the COX enzymes.

My studies in the Ruden laboratory using the Drosophila model system were the first evidence showing that the WNT pathway can be epigenetically regulated [109]. In these studies, we found that mutations in several trithorax-group (TrxG) genes or the *Drosophila* Hsp90 homolog (*Hsp83*) could elicit gain-of-function expression of *wingless* that was epigenetically inherited. The TrxG and polycomb-group genes were the first gene groups to be identified that controlled gene expression through epigenetic mechanisms. Since TrxG genes are responsible for maintenance of active transcription, a mutation in TrxG genes should result in loss of transcription. These results indicate a gene under epigenetic control is involved in repression of the Wnt pathway, since loss of the gene product up-regulates the WNT pathway. A possible explanation of these results surfaced with the discovery that the secreted frizzled-related proteins (SFRPs) are epigenetically regulated [110]. Additionally, SFRP6 was found to be repressed by an epigenetic mechanism by the TrxG gene MLL, which is involved in about 50 different chromosomal translocation in acute leukemia [111]. The SFRPs have been implicated in colorectal cancers and shown to be negatively regulated by DNA methylation early in these cancers [112, 113]. The SFRPs negatively regulate the Wnt pathway by sequestering the ligand in the extracellular matrix. The observations concerning the SFRPs are consistent with our observation that loss-of-function in transcriptional activators (TrxG genes) resulted in gain-of-function in *wingless* expression. In this model loss of epigenetic activation through TrxG genes results in down-regulation of the SFRPs. Lack of sequestration of the ligand due to epigenetic silencing of the SFRPs results in accumulation of the WNT ligand and activated signaling. The impact of these results on oncogenesis is that the microenvironmental influence of SFRP secretion on WNT signaling is epigenetically regulated and possibly influenced by factors that affect epigenetic modulation such as diet [102].

Because leukemia is characterized by ineffective differentiation, constitutive silencing of SFRPs would result in aberrant WNT signaling and promotion of leukemogenesis [13, 102, 114]. This mechanism of promotion of malignancy has been seen in other stem cell related cancers such as colorectal cancers as an early event in pathogenesis [112, 113]. In studies conducted in the Kozak laboratory, they found that genetically identical mice had epigenetic modifications at SFRP5 when fed high fat diets [115]. The extraordinary finding that fatty acids content in the diet can affect SFRP methylation and cause epigenetic effects on obesity has exciting implications in regards to dietary effects through WNT signaling on leukemias.

CONCLUSIONS

The epigenetic suppression of malignancy by inducing differentiation bypasses the genetic aberrations such as chromosomal abnormalities in malignant cells [116, 117]. If these epigenetic events are controllable through dietary interventions or rationally designed compounds of enhanced potency that use the same pathways as these dietary compounds, then a new therapeutic approach to multiple cancer types is possible. The connections between signaling pathways such as WNT to lipid metabolism and epigenetic gene regulation make the exploration of this concept possible in the near future.

REFERENCES

[1]   Gabor Miklos GL, Maleszka R. Epigenomic communication systems in humans and honey bees: From molecules to behavior. Hormones and Behavior 2010.

[2]   Kucharski R, Maleszka J, Foret S, Maleszka R. Nutritional control of reproductive status in honeybees *via* DNA methylation. Science 2008;319(5871): 1827-30.

[3]   Maleszka R. Epigenetic integration of environmental and genomic signals in honey bees: the critical interplay of nutritional, brain and reproductive networks. Epigenetics 2008;3(4): 188-92.

[4]   Rizo A, Vellenga E, de Haan G, Schuringa JJ. Signaling pathways in self-renewing hematopoietic and leukemic stem cells: do all stem cells need a niche? Hum Mol Genet 2006;15 Spec No 2: R210-9.

[5]   Till JE, Mc CE. A direct measurement of the radiation sensitivity of normal mouse bone marrow cells. Radiat Res 1961: 213-22.

[6]   Hayflick L, Moorhead PS. The serial cultivation of human diploid cell strains. Exp Cell Res 1961;25: 585-621.

[7]   Morrison SJ, Uchida N, Weissman IL. The biology of hematopoietic stem cells. Annu Rev Cell Dev Biol 1995;11: 35-71.

[8]   Hanahan D, Weinberg RA. The hallmarks of cancer. Cell 2000;100(1): 57-70.

[9]   Jandl JH. Blood cell formation. Blood:Textbook of Hematology. 2nd ed. New York, NY: Little, Brown and Company; 1996. p. 1-55.

[10]   Morrison SJ, Weissman IL. The long-term repopulating subset of hematopoietic stem cells is deterministic and isolatable by phenotype. Immunity 1994;1(8): 661-73.

[11]   Bonnet D, Dick JE. Human acute myeloid leukemia is organized as a hierarchy that originates from a primitive hematopoietic cell. Nat Med 1997; 3(7): 730-7.

[12]   Hope KJ, Jin L, Dick JE. Acute myeloid leukemia originates from a hierarchy of leukemic stem cell classes that differ in self-renewal capacity. Nat Immunol 2004; 5(7): 738-43.

[13]   Jamieson CH, Ailles LE, Dylla SJ, Muijtjens M, Jones C, Zehnder JL, *et al.* Granulocyte-macrophage progenitors as candidate leukemic stem cells in blast-crisis CML. N Engl J Med 2004; 351(7): 657-67.

[14]   Castor A, Nilsson L, Astrand-Grundstrom I, Buitenhuis M, Ramirez C, Anderson K, *et al.* Distinct patterns of hematopoietic stem cell involvement in acute lymphoblastic leukemia. Nat Med 2005; 11(6): 630-7.

[15]   Krivtsov AV, Twomey D, Feng Z, Stubbs MC, Wang Y, Faber J, *et al.* Transformation from committed progenitor to leukaemia stem cell initiated by MLL-AF9. Nature 2006; 442(7104): 818-22.

[16]   Huntly BJ, Shigematsu H, Deguchi K, Lee BH, Mizuno S, Duclos N, *et al.* MOZ-TIF2, but not BCR-ABL, confers properties of leukemic stem cells to committed murine hematopoietic progenitors. Cancer Cell 2004; 6(6): 587-96.

[17]   Jordan CT. Searching for leukemia stem cells--not yet the end of the road? Cancer Cell 2006; 10(4): 253-4.

[18]   Kuo YH, Landrette SF, Heilman SA, Perrat PN, Garrett L, Liu PP, *et al.* Cbf beta-SMMHC induces distinct abnormal myeloid progenitors able to develop acute myeloid leukemia. Cancer Cell 2006; 9(1): 57-68.

[19]   Feinberg AP, Ohlsson R, Henikoff S. The epigenetic progenitor origin of human cancer. Nat Rev Genet 2006; 7(1): 21-33.

[20]   Meissner A. Epigenetic modifications in pluripotent and differentiated cells. Nat Biotechnol 2010; 28(10): 1079-88.

[21]   Shafa M, Krawetz R, Rancourt DE. Returning to the stem state: epigenetics of recapitulating pre-differentiation chromatin structure. Bioessays 2010; 32(9): 791-9.

[22]   Lotem J, Sachs L. Epigenetics and the plasticity of differentiation in normal and cancer stem cells. Oncogene 2006; 25(59): 7663-72.

[23]   Collas P. Epigenetic states in stem cells. Biochim Biophys Acta 2009; 1790(9): 900-5.

[24]   Fischle W, Wang Y, Allis CD. Histone and chromatin cross-talk. Curr Opin Cell Biol 2003; 15(2): 172-83.

[25]   Turner BM. Cellular memory and the histone code. Cell 2002; 111(3): 285-91.

[26]   Jenuwein T, Allis CD. Translating the histone code. Science 200; 293(5532): 1074-80.

[27]   Cheung P, Allis CD, Sassone-Corsi P. Signaling to chromatin through histone modifications. Cell 2000; 103(2): 263-71.

[28]   Csankovszki G, Panning B, Bates B, Pehrson JR, Jaenisch R. Conditional deletion of Xist disrupts histone macroH2A localization but not maintenance of X inactivation. Nat Genet 1999; 22(4): 323-4.

[29]   Angelov D, Molla A, Perche PY, Hans F, Cote J, Khochbin S, *et al.* The histone variant macroH2A interferes with transcription factor binding and SWI/SNF nucleosome remodeling. Mol Cell 2003; 11(4): 1033-41.

[30]   Meneghini MD, Wu M, Madhani HD. Conserved histone variant H2A.Z protects euchromatin from the ectopic spread of silent heterochromatin. Cell 2007; 112(5): 725-36.

[31]   Hatch CL, Bonner WM. An upstream region of the H2AZ gene promoter modulates promoter activity in different cell types. Biochim Biophys Acta 1996;1305(1-2): 59-62.

[32]   Freitag M, Selker EU. Controlling DNA methylation: many roads to one modification. Curr Opin Genet Dev 2005; 15(2): 191-9.

[33]   De Larco JE, Wuertz BR, Yee D, Rickert BL, Furcht LT. Atypical methylation of the interleukin-8 gene correlates strongly with the metastatic potential of breast carcinoma cells. Proc Natl Acad Sci U S A 2003; 100(24): 13988-93.

[34]   Bird AP, Wolffe AP. Methylation-induced repression--belts, braces, and chromatin. Cell 1999; 99(5): 451-4.

[35]   Bannister AJ, Zegerman P, Partridge JF, Miska EA, Thomas JO, Allshire RC, *et al.* Selective recognition of methylated lysine 9 on histone H3 by the HP1 chromo domain. Nature 2001; 410(6824): 120-4.

[36]   Lachner M, O'Carroll D, Rea S, Mechtler K, Jenuwein T. Methylation of histone H3 lysine 9 creates a binding site for HP1 proteins. Nature 2001; 410(6824): 116-20.

[37]   Paroush Z, Keshet I, Yisraeli J, Cedar H. Dynamics of demethylation and activation of the alpha-actin gene in myoblasts Cell. 1990; 63(6): 1229-37.

[38]   Lubbert M, Brugger W, Mertelsmann R, Kanz L. Developmental regulation of myeloid gene expression and demethylation during *ex vivo* culture of peripheral blood progenitor cells. Blood 1996; 87(2): 447-55.

[39]   Avni O, Rao A. T cell differentiation: a mechanistic view. Curr Opin Immunol 2000; 12(6): 654-9.

[40]   Terskikh AV, Miyamoto T, Chang C, Diatchenko L, Weissman IL. Gene expression analysis of purified hematopoietic stem cells and committed progenitors. Blood 2003; 102(1): 94-101.

[41]   Ringrose L, Paro R. Epigenetic regulation of cellular memory by the Polycomb and Trithorax group proteins. Annu Rev Genet 2004; 38: 413-43.

[42]   Jorgensen HF, Giadrossi S, Casanova M, Endoh M, Koseki H, Brockdorff N, *et al.* Stem cells primed for action: polycomb repressive complexes restrain the expression of lineage-specific regulators in embryonic stem cells. Cell Cycle 2006; 5(13): 1411-4.

[43]   Lessard J, Sauvageau G. Bmi-1 determines the proliferative capacity of normal and leukaemic stem cells. Nature 2003; 423(6937): 255-60.

[44]   Molofsky AV, Pardal R, Iwashita T, Park IK, Clarke MF, Morrison SJ. Bmi-1 dependence distinguishes neural stem cell self-renewal from progenitor proliferation. Nature 2003; 425(6961): 962-7.

[45]   Park IK, Qian D, Kiel M, Becker MW, Pihalja M, Weissman IL, *et al.* Bmi-1 is required for maintenance of adult self-renewing haematopoietic stem cells. Nature 2003; 423(6937): 302-5.

[46]   Bernstein BE, Mikkelsen TS, Xie X, Kamal M, Huebert DJ, Cuff J, *et al.* A Bivalent Chromatin Structure Marks Key Developmental Genes in Embryonic Stem Cells. Cell 2006; 125(2): 315-26.

[47]   Giadrossi S, Dvorkina M, Fisher AG. Chromatin organization and differentiation in embryonic stem cell models. Curr Opin Genet Dev 2007; 17(2): 132-8.

[48]   Azuara V, Perry P, Sauer S, Spivakov M, Jorgensen HF, John RM, *et al.* Chromatin signatures of pluripotent cell lines. Nat Cell Biol 2006; 8(5): 532-8.

[49]   Bernstein BE, Mikkelsen TS, Xie X, Kamal M, Huebert DJ, Cuff J, *et al.* A bivalent chromatin structure marks key developmental genes in embryonic stem cells. Cell 2006; 125(2): 315-26.

[50]   Roh TY, Cuddapah S, Cui K, Zhao K. The genomic landscape of histone modifications in human T cells. Proc Natl Acad Sci U S A 2006; 103(43): 15782-7.

[51]   Mark M, Rijli FM, Chambon P. Homeobox genes in embryogenesis and pathogenesis. Pediatr Res 1997; 42(4): 421-9.

[52]   Blatt C, Aberdam D, Schwartz R, Sachs L. DNA rearrangement of a homeobox gene in myeloid leukaemic cells [published erratum appears in EMBO J 1989 Apr;8(4):1288]. Embo J 1988; 7(13): 4283-90.

[53]   Perkins A, Kongsuwan K, Visvader J, Adams JM, Cory S. Homeobox gene expression plus autocrine growth factor production elicits myeloid leukemia. Proc Natl Acad Sci U S A 1990; 87(21): 8398-402.

[54]   Hatano M, Roberts CW, Minden M, Crist WM, Korsmeyer SJ. Deregulation of a homeobox gene, HOX11, by the t(10;14) in T cell leukemia. Science 1991; 253(5015): 79-82.

[55]   Sauvageau G, Thorsteinsdottir U, Hough MR, Hugo P, Lawrence HJ, Largman C, *et al.* Overexpression of HOXB3 in hematopoietic cells causes defective lymphoid development and progressive myeloproliferation. Immunity 1997; 6(1): 13-22.

[56]   Kroon E, Krosl J, Thorsteinsdottir U, Baban S, Buchberg AM, Sauvageau G. Hoxa9 transforms primary bone marrow cells through specific collaboration with Meis1a but not Pbx1b. Embo J 1998; 17(13): 3714-25.

[57]   Thorsteinsdottir U, Sauvageau G, Humphries RK. Hox homeobox genes as regulators of normal and leukemic hematopoiesis. Hematol Oncol Clin North Am 1997; 11(6): 1221-37.

[58]   Borrow J, Shearman AM, Stanton VP, Jr., Becher R, Collins T, Williams AJ, *et al.* The t(7;11)(p15;p15) translocation in acute myeloid leukaemia fuses the genes for nucleoporin NUP98 and class I homeoprotein HOXA9. Nat Genet 1996; 12(2): 159-67.

[59]   Moskow JJ, Bullrich F, Huebner K, Daar IO, Buchberg AM. Meis1, a PBX1-related homeobox gene involved in myeloid leukemia in BXH-2 mice. Mol Cell Biol 1995; 15(10): 5434-43.

[60]   Lasa A, Carnicer MJ, Aventin A, Estivill C, Brunet S, Sierra J, *et al.* MEIS 1 expression is downregulated through promoter hypermethylation in AML1-ETO acute myeloid leukemias. Leukemia 2004 Jul; 18(7): 1231-7.

[61]   Zion M, Ben-Yehuda D, Avraham A, Cohen O, Wetzler M, Melloul D, *et al.* Progressive *de novo* DNA methylation at the bcr-abl locus in the course of chronic myelogenous leukemia. Proc Natl Acad Sci U S A 1994; 91(22): 10722-6.

[62]   Issa JP, Kantarjian H, Mohan A, O'Brien S, Cortes J, Pierce S, *et al.* Methylation of the ABL1 promoter in chronic myelogenous leukemia: lack of prognostic significance. Blood 1999; 93(6): 2075-80.

[63]   Ge XQ, Tanaka K, Mansyur A, Tazawa H, Iwato K, Kyo T, *et al.* Possible prediction of myeloid and lymphoid crises in chronic myelocytic leukemia at onset by determining the methylation status of the major breakpoint cluster region. Cancer Genet Cytogenet 2001; 126(2): 102-10.

[64]   Nguyen TT, Mohrbacher AF, Tsai YC, Groffen J, Heisterkamp N, Nichols PW, *et al.* Quantitative measure of c-abl and p15 methylation in chronic myelogenous leukemia: biological implications. Blood 2000; 95(9): 2990-2.

[65]   Quesnel B, Guillerm G, Vereecque R, Wattel E, Preudhomme C, Bauters F, *et al.* Methylation of the p15(INK4b) gene in myelodysplastic syndromes is frequent and acquired during disease progression. Blood 1998; 91(8): 2985-90.

[66]   Mizuno S, Chijiwa T, Okamura T, Akashi K, Fukumaki Y, Niho Y, *et al.* Expression of DNA methyltransferases DNMT1, 3A, and 3B in normal hematopoiesis and in acute and chronic myelogenous leukemia. Blood 2001; 97(5): 1172-9.

[67]   Sved J, Bird A. The expected equilibrium of the CpG dinucleotide in vertebrate genomes under a mutation model. Proc Natl Acad Sci U S A 1990; 87(12): 4692-6.

[68]   Schoch C, Kern W, Schnittger S, Hiddemann W, Haferlach T. Karyotype is an independent prognostic parameter in therapy-related acute myeloid leukemia (t-AML): an analysis of 93 patients with t-AML in comparison to 1091 patients with *de novo* AML. Leukemia 2004; 18(1): 120-5.

[69]   Ekmekci CG, Gutierrez MI, Siraj AK, Ozbek U, Bhatia K. Aberrant methylation of multiple tumor suppressor genes in acute myeloid leukemia. Am J Hematol 2004; 77(3): 233-40.

[70]   Feher I, Gidali J. Prostaglandin E2 as stimulator of haemopoietic stem cell proliferation. Nature. 1974 Feb 22;247(442):550-1.

[71]   Gidali J, Feher I. The effect of E type prostaglandins on the proliferation of haemopoietic stem cells *in vivo*. Cell Tissue Kinet 1977; 10(4): 365-73.

[72]   Williams N. Preferential inhibition of murine macrophage colony formation by prostaglandin E. Blood 1979; 53(6): 1089-94.

[73]   Pelus LM, Broxmeyer HE, Kurland JI, Moore MA. Regulation of macrophage and granulocyte proliferation. Specificities of prostaglandin E and lactoferrin. J Exp Med 1979;150(2): 277-92.

[74]   Verma DS, Spitzer G, Zander AR, McCredie KB, Dicke KA. Prostaglandin E1-mediated augmentation of human granulocyte-macrophage progenitor cell growth *in vitro*. Leuk Res 1981; 5(1): 65-71.

[75]   Pelus LM. Association between colony forming units-granulocyte macrophage expression of Ia-like (HLA-DR) antigen and control of granulocyte and macrophage production. A new role for prostaglandin E. J Clin Invest 1982; 70(3): 568-78.

[76]   Lord AM, North TE, Zon LI. Prostaglandin E2: making more of your marrow. Cell Cycle 2007; 6(24): 3054-7.

[77]   Frisch BJ, Porter RL, Gigliotti BJ, Olm-Shipman AJ, Weber JM, O'Keefe RJ, *et al. In vivo* prostaglandin E2 treatment alters the bone marrow microenvironment and preferentially expands short-term hematopoietic stem cells. Blood 2009; 114(19): 4054-63.

[78]   North TE, Goessling W, Walkley CR, Lengerke C, Kopani KR, Lord AM, *et al.* Prostaglandin E2 regulates vertebrate haematopoietic stem cell homeostasis. Nature 2007; 447(7147): 1007-11.

[79]   Hoggatt J, Singh P, Sampath J, Pelus LM. Prostaglandin E2 enhances hematopoietic stem cell homing, survival, and proliferation. Blood 2009; 113(22): 5444-55.

[80]   Lorenz M, Slaughter HS, Wescott DM, Carter SI, Schnyder B, Dinchuk JE, *et al.* Cyclooxygenase-2 is essential for normal recovery from 5-fluorouracil-induced myelotoxicity in mice. Exp Hematol 1999; 27(10): 1494-502.

[81]   Dupuis F, Desplat V, Praloran V, Denizot Y. Effects of lipidic mediators on the growth of human myeloid and erythroid marrow progenitors. J Lipid Mediat Cell Signal 1997; 16(3): 117-25.

[82]   Rocca B, Spain LM, Pure E, Langenbach R, Patrono C, FitzGerald GA. Distinct roles of prostaglandin H synthases 1 and 2 in T-cell development. J Clin Invest 1999; 103(10): 1469-77.

[83]   Rocca B, FitzGerald GA. Cyclooxygenases and prostaglandins: shaping up the immune response. Int Immunopharmacol 2002; 2(5): 603-30.

[84]   Villablanca EJ, Pistocchi A, Court FA, Cotelli F, Bordignon C, Allende ML, *et al.* Abrogation of prostaglandin E2/EP4 signaling impairs the development of rag1+ lymphoid precursors in the thymus of zebrafish embryos. J Immunol 2007; 179(1): 357-64.

[85]   Hoff T, DeWitt D, Kaever V, Resch K, Goppelt-Struebe M. Differentiation-associated expression of prostaglandin G/H synthase in monocytic cells. FEBS Lett 1993; 320(1): 38-42.

[86]   Smith CJ, Morrow JD, Roberts LJ, 2nd, Marnett LJ. Differentiation of monocytoid THP-1 cells with phorbol ester induces expression of prostaglandin endoperoxide synthase-1 (COX-1). Biochem Biophys Res Commun 1993; 192(2): 787-93.

[87]   Williams N, Jackson H. Limitation of macrophage production in long-term marrow cultures containing prostaglandin E. J Cell Physiol 1980; 103(2): 239-46.

[88]   Miura GI, Treisman JE. Lipid modification of secreted signaling proteins. Cell Cycle 2006; 5(11): 1184-8.

[89]   Li D, Ng A, Mann NJ, Sinclair AJ. Contribution of meat fat to dietary arachidonic acid. Lipids 1998; 33(4): 437-40.

[90]   Hagve TA, Christophersen BO. Effect of dietary fats on arachidonic acid and eicosapentaenoic acid biosynthesis and conversion to C22 fatty acids in isolated rat liver cells. Biochim Biophys Acta 1984; 796(2): 205-17.

[91]   Rose DP, Connolly JM. Omega-3 fatty acids as cancer chemopreventive agents. Pharmacol Ther 1999;83(3): 217-44.

[92]   Germain E, Lavandier F, Chajes V, Schubnel V, Bonnet P, Lhuillery C, *et al.* Dietary n-3 polyunsaturated fatty acids and oxidants increase rat mammary tumor sensitivity to epirubicin without change in cardiac toxicity. Lipids 1999; 34 Suppl: S203.

[93]   Hardman WE, Barnes CJ, Knight CW, Cameron IL. Effects of iron supplementation and ET-18-OCH3 on MDA-MB 231 breast carcinomas in nude mice consuming a fish oil diet. Br J Cancer 1997; 76(3): 347-54.

[94]   Karmali RA. Historical perspective and potential use of n-3 fatty acids in therapy of cancer cachexia. Nutrition 1996;12(1 Suppl): S2-4.

[95]   Oberley LW, Spitz DR. Assay of superoxide dismutase activity in tumor tissue. Methods Enzymol 1984; 105: 457-64.

[96]   Varney ME, Hardman WE, Sollars VE. Omega 3 fatty acids reduce myeloid progenitor cell frequency in the bone marrow of mice and promote progenitor cell differentiation. Lipids Health Dis 2009; 8:9.

[97]   Varney ME, Buchanan JT, Dementieva Y, Elaine Hardman W, Sollars VE. A High Omega-3 Fatty Acid Diet has Different Effects on Early and Late Stage Myeloid Progenitors. Lipids 2011; 46(1): 47-57.

[98]   Foret S, Kucharski R, Pittelkow Y, Lockett GA, Maleszka R. Epigenetic regulation of the honey bee transcriptome: unravelling the nature of methylated genes. BMC Genomics 2009; 10: 472.

[99]   Cadigan KM, Nusse R. Wnt signaling: a common theme in animal development. Genes Dev 1997; 11(24): 3286-305.

[100]   Reya T, Duncan AW, Ailles L, Domen J, Scherer DC, Willert K, *et al.* A role for Wnt signalling in self-renewal of haematopoietic stem cells. Nature 2003; 423(6938): 409-14.

[101]   Trowbridge JJ, Xenocostas A, Moon RT, Bhatia M. Glycogen synthase kinase-3 is an *in vivo* regulator of hematopoietic stem cell repopulation. Nat Med 2006; 12(1): 89-98.

[102]   Sollars VE. The epigenomic viewpoint on cellular differentiation of myeloid progenitor cells as it pertains to leukemogenesis. Current Genomics 2005; 6(3): 137-44.

[103]   Willert K, Brown JD, Danenberg E, Duncan AW, Weissman IL, Reya T, *et al.* Wnt proteins are lipid-modified and can act as stem cell growth factors. Nature 2003; 423(6938): 448-52.

[104]   Castellone MD, Teramoto H, Williams BO, Druey KM, Gutkind JS. Prostaglandin E2 promotes colon cancer cell growth through a Gs-axin-beta-catenin signaling axis. Science 2005; 310(5753): 1504-10.

[105]   Giardiello FM, Yang VW, Hylind LM, Krush AJ, Petersen GM, Trimbath JD, *et al.* Primary chemoprevention of familial adenomatous polyposis with sulindac. N Engl J Med 2002; 346(14): 1054-9.

[106]   Shao J, Jung C, Liu C, Sheng H. Prostaglandin E2 Stimulates the beta-catenin/T cell factor-dependent transcription in colon cancer. J Biol Chem 2005; 280(28): 26565-72.

[107]   Goessling W, North TE, Loewer S, Lord AM, Lee S, Stoick-Cooper CL, *et al.* Genetic interaction of PGE2 and Wnt signaling regulates developmental specification of stem cells and regeneration. Cell 2009; 136(6): 1136-47.

[108]   Lim K, Han C, Xu L, Isse K, Demetris AJ, Wu T. Cyclooxygenase-2-derived prostaglandin E2 activates beta-catenin in human cholangiocarcinoma cells: evidence for inhibition of these signaling pathways by omega 3 polyunsaturated fatty acids. Cancer Res 2008; 68(2): 553-60.

[109]   Sollars V, Lu X, Xiao L, Wang X, Garfinkel MD, Ruden DM. Evidence for an epigenetic mechanism by which Hsp90 acts as a capacitor for morphological evolution. Nat Genet 2003; 33(1): 70-4.

[110]   Rattner A, Hsieh JC, Smallwood PM, Gilbert DJ, Copeland NG, Jenkins NA, *et al.* A family of secreted proteins contains homology to the cysteine-rich ligand-binding domain of frizzled receptors. Proc Natl Acad Sci U S A 1997; 94(7): 2859-63.

[111]   Schraets D, Lehmann T, Dingermann T, Marschalek R. MLL-mediated transcriptional gene regulation investigated by gene expression profiling. Oncogene 2003; 22(23): 3655-68.

[112]   Caldwell GM, Jones C, Gensberg K, Jan S, Hardy RG, Byrd P, *et al.* The Wnt antagonist sFRP1 in colorectal tumorigenesis. Cancer Res 2004; 64(3): 883-8.

[113]   Suzuki H, Watkins DN, Jair KW, Schuebel KE, Markowitz SD, Dong Chen W, *et al.* Epigenetic inactivation of SFRP genes allows constitutive WNT signaling in colorectal cancer. Nat Genet 2004; 36(4): 417-22.

[114]   Wang GG, Pasillas MP, Kamps MP. Meis1 programs transcription of FLT3 and cancer stem cell character, using a mechanism that requires interaction with Pbx and a novel function of the Meis1 C-terminus. Blood 2005; 106(1): 254-64.

[115]   Koza RA, Nikonova L, Hogan J, Rim JS, Mendoza T, Faulk C, *et al.* Changes in gene expression foreshadow diet-induced obesity in genetically identical mice. PLoS Genet 2006; 2(5): e81.

[116]   Sachs L. Cell differentiation and bypassing of genetic defects in the suppression of malignancy. Cancer Res 1987; 47(8): 1981-6.

[117]   Sachs L. The Wellcome Foundation lecture, 1986. The molecular regulators of normal and leukaemic blood cells. Proc R Soc Lond B Biol Sci 1987; 231(1264): 289-312.

CHAPTER 7

Nutrition, Oxidative Stress and Cancer

Monica Valentovic[*] and Nalini Santanam

Nutrition and Cancer Center, Department of Pharmacology, Physiology & Toxicology, Joan C. Edwards School of Medicine, Marshall University, Huntington, WV, USA

Abstract: Phytochemicals are now increasingly being used as nutritional supplements to either prevent or treat chronic diseases including cancer. The mechanisms of action of the phytochemicals can range from: inhibiting oxidative stress, apoptosis, inhibiting mitochondrial damage and inhibiting or promoting angiogenesis. The significance of oxidative stress in the etiology of aging and several chronic diseases: including cardiovascular disease, cancer and Alzheimer's, has given support to the usage of these phytochemicals to inhibit oxidative damage. The complexity of the chemistry involved in oxidative stress damage to cells or tissue adds to the consideration of choice of the phytochemical to combat these effects. Cancer is a multifactorial disease. Epidemiological studies have shown beneficial effects of several phytochemicals in the prevention and treatment of several types of cancer. This chapter will address the role of oxidative stress in cancer and the antioxidant action of some of the most popularly used phytochemicals including-green tea, soy, resveratrol and ellagic acid (flavonoids, polyphenols).

Keywords: Diet, Ellagic Acid, Food, Green Tea, JNK, NADPH, Phytochemical, Reactive Oxygen Species, Prostate Specific Antigen, Resveratrol, Soy.

INTRODUCTION

Cancer is a major health concern as it is the second leading cause of death in the United States [1]. Excess oxygen radicals have been associated with cancer and other diseases such as cardiovascular disease and aging [2, 3]. Oxidative stress occurs when the cellular balance between pro-oxidant and antioxidant systems shift towards a pro-oxidant milieu. Reactive oxygen species (ROS) include the non-radical hydrogen peroxide as well as the free radicals: superoxide anion and hydroxyl radical. Normal cellular functions such as cytochrome P450 drug metabolism, mitochondrial respiration, neutrophil phagocytosis, activation of macrophages and hepatic Kupffer cell function all generate ROS. Oxidative stress and generation of ROS serves an important role in normal function and in disease conditions [4]. For example, hydrogen peroxide (H_2O_2) is needed in normal thyroid hormone synthesis while excess levels of oxygen species occurring in hemachromatosis are toxic to the liver.

Mitochondrial respiration and activity of the electron transport chain result in a steady source of oxygen radicals (Fig. **1**), specifically superoxide anion, from molecular oxygen [5, 6]. Superoxide anion is then converted by superoxide dismutase to hydrogen peroxide and water. Hydrogen peroxide is highly toxic since it is uncharged and can readily enter a cell unless it is detoxified. In the presence of transition metals such as iron, hydrogen peroxide can be converted non-enzymatically to more toxic hydroxyl radical by the Fenton and Haber-Weiss reactions. Excess formation of ROS can result in damage to cell membranes, peroxidation of lipids and interact with DNA and proteins to alter normal cell function.

ROS are not formed exclusively by the mitochondria, as oxygen species are found in other intracellular sites such as the: smooth endoplasmic reticulum, cytosol and phagosomes. Normal phagocytic action of neutrophils on bacteria requires conversion of oxygen to superoxide and hydrogen peroxide by NADPH (Nicotinamide Adenine Dinucleotide Phosphate) oxidase. The activation of NADPH oxidase, a membrane bound enzyme, results in a burst of ROS formation [7]. Neutrophil phagocytic action further utilizes

---

*Address Correspondence to Monica Valentovic: Nutrition and Cancer Center, Department of Pharmacology, Physiology and Toxicology, Joan C. Edwards School of Medicine, Marshall University, Byrd Biotechnology Science Center, Room 435G, 1700 Third Avenue, Huntington WV, 25755, USA; E-mail: valentov@marshall.edu

Pier Paolo Claudio and Richard M. Niles (Eds)

hydrogen peroxide and myeloperoxidase to generate hypochlorous acid to destroy bacteria. Chronic granulomatous disease is an inherited condition where neutrophils lack NADPH oxidase causing an increased susceptibility to infection, since these neutrophils generate insufficient levels of ROS. Intracellular ROS products can have extracellular impact such as vascular endothelial cell ROS products causing oxidation of low-density lipoprotein (LDL) particles and contributing toward the progression of atherosclerosis. More recent studies have indicated that ROS are second messengers that are capable of altering cellular signaling for apoptosis. ROS activates c-Jun N-terminal kinase (JNK) and promotes apoptosis by breaking the inhibitory interaction of glutathione S-transferase (GST) pi with JNK [8, 9]. ROS can oxidize available cysteine within a protein and modify protein function. Oxidation of cysteine in thioredoxin causes dissociation with apoptosis signaling kinase 1 (ASK1) resulting in ASK1 activation and prolonged activation of JNK [8].

Detoxification of ROS is normally regulated by several enzymatic pathways within the cell. ROS can be rapidly detoxified by cellular antioxidant enzymes such as, superoxide dismutase, glutathione peroxidase and catalase [9-12]. Superoxide dismutases (SOD) (manganese SOD, copper-Zinc SOD) are located either in the mitochondria or cytosol and are responsible for the conversion of superoxide anion to hydrogen peroxide. Glutathione peroxidase along with reduced glutathione (GSH) is responsible for detoxification of hydrogen peroxide. Glutathione peroxidase, located within the mitochondria and cytosol, oxidizes GSH to glutathione disulfide (GSSG) which is then reduced by one electron addition back to reduced GSH by the enzyme GSSG reductase. Catalase converts hydrogen peroxide rapidly to oxygen and is readily present in red blood cells (Fig. **1**). In addition to these cellular antioxidants, there are several other natural antioxidants both from plant and animal sources that can quench ROS and these have been studied for their beneficial effects in cardiovascular disease and cancer [13-15].

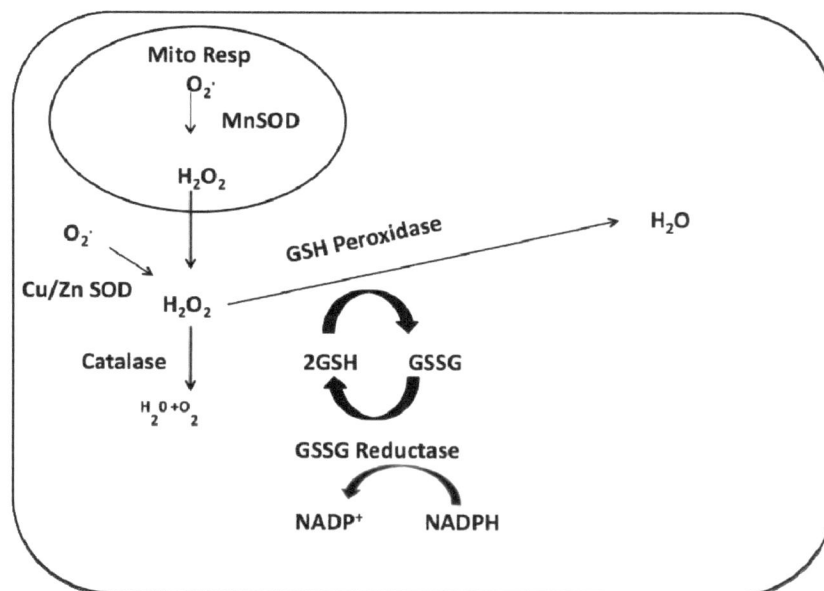

Figure 1: Cellular Detoxification pathways. Superoxide anion (O_2^-) is converted by manganese superoxide (MnSOD) and copper/zinc SOD to hydrogen peroxide (H_2O_2). Hydrogen peroxide is converted to water and oxygen by catalase. Glutathione (GSH) peroxidase can also detoxify H_2O_2 to water by oxidation of GSH to glutathione disulfide (GSSG). GSSG is reduced to GSH by glutathione (GSSG) reductase in the presence of NADPH.

Cancer cells are associated with higher oxidative stress due to increased cell activity and alterations in mitochondrial activity [2, 16]. Early evidence of the role of oxidative stress in cancer came from studies where normal cells were transformed when exposed to reactive oxygen species [17]. High levels of hydrogen peroxide (H_2O_2) are produced spontaneously by some cancer cells [18]. Human colon, melanoma, neuroblastoma and ovarian cancer cell lines generated H_2O_2 at a rate of 0.2-0.7 nmol $H_2O_2/10^4$ cells/h [18]. The levels of H_2O_2 production was very high relative to phorbol ester stimulated neutrophils that generated 1.4 nmol $H_2O_2/10^4$ cells/h when assayed simultaneously with the cancer cells. In addition, another oxygen radical, superoxide anion was also spontaneously generated in high quantities by human melanoma cell lines SK-Mel 23, 28, 30, and 131 and human colon carcinoma cell line HT 29. These findings demonstrate that certain cancer cells have spontaneously higher levels of oxygen radicals compared to noncancerous cells although the mechanism has yet to be established for the increased oxygen radical generation. These initial studies led to over seven thousand publications to date, that have reported on the link between cancer and oxidative stress. Depending on the concentrations of the ROS it can either inhibit tumor growth or promote it. Excess ROS generation can oxidatively modify DNA (8-hydroxy guanosine-8-OHdG) or cause DNA misrepair and genomic instability. Prolonged or excess ROS generation can induce DNA alterations that promote tumor cancer formation. Unfortunately, tumor cells have decreased antioxidant defense which shifts the cellular balance towards increased oxidative stress.

Natural products that can modify ROS levels may be of benefit in prevention of cancer development. Natural products are also a potential source of active compounds that may have a beneficial role in reducing oxidative stress in cancer cells [19-21]. Natural products are a group of compounds that are structurally diverse and identification of the active components is a daunting task. However, detection of active agents that could have beneficial effects in modulating cancer cell proliferation is of clinical significance. In this chapter we describe the uses of few of the natural products tested for cancer prevention. It should be noted that there several other phytochemicals that are also being tested for their beneficial effects in cancer or cardiovascular disease prevention.

ELLAGIC ACID

Pomegranate fruit and its juice are a rich source of polyphenols. The most common polyphenols in pomegranate juice are ellagitannins [22]. Other sources of ellagitannins include muscadine grapes, walnuts and many berries especially strawberries, raspberries and cranberries. Ellagitannins are hydrolyzed in an aqueous environment to release ellagic acid. This polyphenol has been suggested to have potential anticancer beneficial effects. Evidence also exists in the literature to suggest that ellagic acid possesses cardioprotective properties. These cardioprotective effects are related to the antioxidant activity of the ellagitannins. A 25 μM concentration of ellagic acid inhibits the oxidation of the principal cholesterol carrier in plasma, low density lipoproteins (LDL). Oxidized lipids are toxic to endothelial cells and can induce endothelial cell death in culture. Ellagic acid slowed LDL oxidation with an IC50 of 20 μM and this antioxidant property would be beneficial for cardioprotection [23] and cancer.

Ellagic acid may have beneficial anticancer effects based on a clinical study in male prostate cancer patients [24]. Prostate specific antigen (PSA) doubling time was prolonged in men with prostate cancer by daily ingestion of just 8 ounces of pomegranate juice. PSA doubling time went from 15 months to 54 months following pomegranate juice ingestion [25]. Pomegranate ingestion was well tolerated by all study subjects and was not associated with any significant side effects. Additional studies by these investigators showed that pomegranate treatment *in vivo* slowed tumor expression and growth of LAPC-4 human prostate cancer cells in immune-compromised SCID mice [26]. Pomegranate juice slowed tumor growth beginning at 2 weeks of treatment and tumor growth was 50% of tumors in untreated mice after 4 weeks of oral administration of pomegranate extract. The anticancer action of pomegranate may differ between *in vivo* administrations compared to *in vitro*. *In vivo,* ellagic acid is converted in the intestinal tract by gut flora to urolithin A, which is absorbed at sufficiently high levels to be detected in plasma [26]. These authors also observed that urolithin A was more potent than ellagic acid for inhibition of tumor cell growth when added *in vitro* to cancer cell lines. Further studies will be needed to determine the relative contributions of ellagic acid and urolithin A to the anticancer properties of pomegranate.

The mechanism for ellagic acid anticancer effects is not entirely known. Ellagic acid does not appear to inhibit the tumor producing activity of polychlorinated biphenyls (PCB), which is thought to be associated with induction of oxidative stress. Rats provided with ellagic acid supplemented rodent chow failed to show any reduction in liver tumors following treatment with PCBs [27]. Ellagic acid (100 μM) does appear to reduce oxidative DNA damage induced by 4-hydroxy-17ß-estradiol [28] as detected by monitoring the formation of 8-oxodeoxyguanosine. Feeding 400 ppm ellagic acid in the diet also reduced oxidative DNA adducts in the liver of mice, which suggests that sufficient amounts of ellagic acid were absorbed to mediate this anti oxidant effect. Gene expression profiling analysis indicated that ellagic acid feeding upregulated DNA repair enzymes that may be a unique mechanism to reduce cancer growth by ellagic acid [29, 30]. Further studies are needed to assess the various mechanisms responsible for ellagic acid's anticancer activity.

GREEN TEA

Green tea contains numerous polyphenols including: epigallocatechin-3-gallate (EGCG), epicatechin (EC), epigallocatechin (EGC) and epicatechin-3-gallate (ECG). Drinking green tea or ingestion of dietary supplements containing green tea components has shown promise in human clinical studies in patients with cancer [31]. Consumption of green tea extract supplement, equivalent to drinking more than 10 cups of green tea daily, reduced the recurrence of colorectal cancer in Japanese men [31].

In men, prostate cancer is one of the leading causes of mortality associated with cancer [32]. In a clinical study, men with prostate cancer ingested a supplement called Polyphenon E, containing 1.3 g of green tea polyphenols which included 800 mg of EGCG prior to prostatectomy [33]. Polyphenon E reduced plasma levels of prostate-specific antigen (PSA), hepatocyte growth factor (HGF) and vascular endothelial growth factor (VEGF) when compared to plasma levels prior to treatment. Polyphenon E treatment in addition to decreasing HGF did not increase plasma liver enzymes.

EGCG (MW 458.37) arrests human prostate cancer cell growth as a function of concentration. A 40-80 µg/ml concentration (87 µM) of EGCG arrested human prostate cancer cell line growth in hormone-sensitive LNCaP cells and hormone-insensitive DU-145 cells. Maximal growth inhibition was also time-dependent with maximum effect occurring within 48 h [34-37]. The action of green tea polyphenols was further enhanced by inhibition of cyclo-oxygenase isozymes 1 and 2 using the non-steroidal anti-inflammatory inhibitor ibuprofen [33, 37]. Testosterone-insensitive DU-145 cell growth inhibition was improved by co-addition of 40 µg/ml EGCG and 1 mM ibuprofen, to inhibit cyclo-oxygenase enzymes [38]. The mechanism for EGCG inhibition of growth may be related to oxidative stress and activation of the caspase pathway [39, 40]. EGCG activated the caspase pathway as caspase 9 activity was elevated in the DU-145 cells treated with EGCG, resulting in apoptosis.

The action of EGCG on oxidative stress is dependent on its concentration. A 100 µM concentration of EGCG added to human MIA PaCa-2 pancreatic cancer cells induced a burst in ROS [41]. EGCG induced apoptosis in MIA PaCa-2 pancreatic cancer cells beginning at a concentration of 100 µM. Interestingly, the induction of apoptosis and ROS generation was blocked by co-incubation with the glutathione synthesis precursor, N-acetylcysteine [42]. These finding strongly suggest that the action of EGCG to induce apoptosis and decrease tumor cell proliferation are related to induction of ROS.

RESVERATROL

Resveratrol (RES) or *trans*-3,4′5-trihydroxystilbene, is a polyphenolic phytoalexin found in the skin of grapes, red wine, Japanese Knotweed, nuts and mulberries. Phytoalexins are agents produced by plants to impede antimicrobial or antifungal growth; RES is generated to reduce powdery mildew infestation of grapes. RES exists in the *cis* and *trans* conformation and the *trans* isomer can be converted by UV light to the *cis* conformation. RES is generated within the skin of grapes following exposure of the plant to growing conditions favoring fungal growth. Variability in growing conditions and fungal development of powdery mildew will result in variability in RES content of the same grape varieties depending on geographic location of the grapes.

Moderate red wine ingestion was reported in 1992 to reduce cardiovascular disease and referred to this habit as the *French Paradox* [43]. Red wine contains RES as well as many structurally diverse chemicals that contribute toward their cardioprotective effects. More recent studies by various laboratories have examined the beneficial effect of RES in cancer. RES possesses anticancer properties against some types of carcinoma. The potential mechanisms for RES anti-cancer action have been proposed to include: antioxidant activity, modulation of cell cycle-regulating proteins and induction of apoptosis in multiple carcinoma cell lines [44-46].

RES reduced cell growth and proliferation of two human ovarian cancer cell lines, A2780 and CaOV3 and in a murine xenograft model [47, 48]. RES alters all 3 stages of tumor development and has been shown to slow tumor initiation, tumor promotion and growth of breast cancer cells [49-51]. The significance of this finding is that RES possesses anticancer properties at least when added to cultured cancer cells. A more critical question for clinical relevance is whether RES can be protective *in vivo*. Studies using a xenograft mouse model treated with breast cancer cells reported that RES reduced breast cancer cell development and tumor size in the xenograft mouse model, suggesting that sufficient RES levels can be attained *in vivo* to elicit a potential therapeutic effect [52].

A key question for all natural products is the mechanism of action for the observed protective effects. Potential mechanisms of action for RES anti-cancer properties have included: activation of apoptosis, inhibition of angiogenesis and oxidative stress [45, 46]. RES has been reported to reduce oxidative stress both *in vitro* and *in vivo* in humans. RES addition to human platelet suspensions *in vitro* reduced oxidative stress [53]. RES addition in the concentration range of 25-100 μM reduced protein carbonyl formation, a marker of oxidative stress, when platelets were stressed by incubation with peroxynitrite.

In vivo ingestion of wine has also been shown to provide sufficient levels of RES to alter oxidative stress in human platelets. Gresele and associates [54] had volunteers ingest 300 ml/day red or white wine for 15 days and noted a higher level of nitric oxide in platelets collected at the end of the 15 day period. Gresesle *et al.* further noted that RES ingestions reduced the pro-inflammatory marker, p38 mitogen-activated protein kinase (p38MAPK) and was associated with a decreased activity of NADPH oxidase, a source of intracellular ROS. A decrease in NADPH oxidase would further support the notion that RES reduced pro-inflammatory activators which may also aid in its anti-cancer role.

Other enzymatic pathways have also been reported to be modified by RES and may have an important role in reducing oxidative stress. As mentioned earlier, SOD is an important enzyme in dismutation of superoxide anion. RES may increase SOD activity, which would be beneficial in reducing the levels of ROS within the cell. Robb and associates [55] noted that MnSOD enzymatic activity and protein expression were increased in normal human fibroblast MRC-5 cells following 2 weeks exposure to RES. The effect of RES on SOD was unique to mitochondrial MnSOD, as Cu/Zn SOD protein expression and activity were not induced. RES stimulation of MnSOD protein expression was time dependent as activation of MnSOD protein expression was increased 3 and 6 fold above control (0 μM RES) at 72 h and 2 weeks, respectively; the extent of protein expression was similar at all time periods for cells exposed to 50 and 100 μM RES. The increase in protein expression was associated with increased MnSOD enzyme activity as MnSOD activity was increased 13 fold by 2 week exposure to 50 μM RES. The increase in MnSOD would facilitate a reduction in mitochondrial superoxide. The early steps in the initiation of apoptosis by RES still needs to be better understood. RES has a concentration and time dependent tumor killing action on breast cancer cells that is both dependent and independent of caspase 3. RES (25-200 μM) exhibited antitumor activity with a comparable IC50 of 129 and 152 μM for MDA-MB-231 and MCF-7 breast cancer cells, respectively [56]. These findings are interesting since MCF-7 cells lack a functioning caspase-3. The mechanism for induction of apoptosis in MCF-7 and MDA-MB-231 cells when exposed to RES was mediated by a dissipation of the mitochondrial membrane potential, activation of mitochondrial alterations in Ca^{2+}-activated proteases, stimulating a rise in intracellular calcium from the endoplasmic reticulum. MDA-MB-231 cells additionally activated caspases-3 and 9 which would induce apoptosis through the mitochondrial intrinsic pathway. Based on these results, the effects of RES are complicated as it is apparent that RES exerts its anti-tumor effects through multiple pathways. Recent reports provide strong evidence that RES also possess pro-oxidant activity in certain conditions [58, 59]. DNA degradation in human lymphocytes was initiated by a combined exposure to RES in the presence of copper (II). The presence of copper (II) was critical since RES alone did not induce DNA degradation. DNA degradation within human lymphocytes occurred when lymphocytes were incubated with the combination of 20 μM copper (II) and 50 μM RES [58]. Addition of copper chelators, prevented DNA degradation within lymphocytes by the combination of copper and RES while iron chelators had no effect [59]. The potential clinical relevance is that copper levels are higher in the serum and tumor for certain cancers such as breast and prostate [59]. Future studies will need to address whether the pro-oxidant action of RES in the presence of copper can be developed as a potential chemotherapeutic delivery.

SOY

Soybean products are a staple diet in several of the Asian countries including, China and Japan. The major phytochemicals associated with soy and those that are studied for their health promoting properties are the isoflavones, genistein and daidzein (Fig. **2**) [57, 58]. Due to their similarity in structure to estrogens and since they harbor a weak estrogen-like activity, genistein (5, 7, 4'-trihydroxyisoflavone) and daidzein (7,4'-dihydroxyisoflavone) are considered to be phytoestrogens. Epidemiological studies do show several health benefits such as lower cardiovascular disease, diabetes and a lower incidence of prostate, colon and breast cancer with soy consumption. In the United States, the FDA has suggested that 25 mg soy consumption daily is beneficial to health [59].

Genistein and other soy isoflavones have anti-oxidant and other cellular protective effects [60]. Early studies on the beneficial effects of soy isoflavones were conflicting. For example there are studies that question the anti-apoptotic effects of soy isoflavones. While genistein has been shown to have an anti-apoptotic activity by protecting BCL-2 from damage by t-butylhydroperoxide treatment in human cortical neuronal cells (HCN1 and HCN2) [61], there are other reports that show a pro-apoptotic activity of genistein in PC12 cells [62]. Also, since studies have shown that genistein and/or daidzein induces cancers in reproductive organs in rodents, such as the uterus and vulva [60], there is considerable controversy whether soy products are protective against recurrence in women with successfully treated breast cancer.

However, there are a number of studies that document the antioxidant properties of genistein and to a lesser extent other soy isoflavones raising the possibility that these compounds could have anti-apoptotic properties. In cell culture studies, genistein exerts its anti-cancer effects through various pathways. For example, in breast (MCF7, MDA-MD-231) and prostate cancer cells (PC3), genistein induces apoptosis by activating Bcl-2 and down-regulating Bax. Genistein also causes cell-cycle arrest in breast and prostate cancer cells [63].

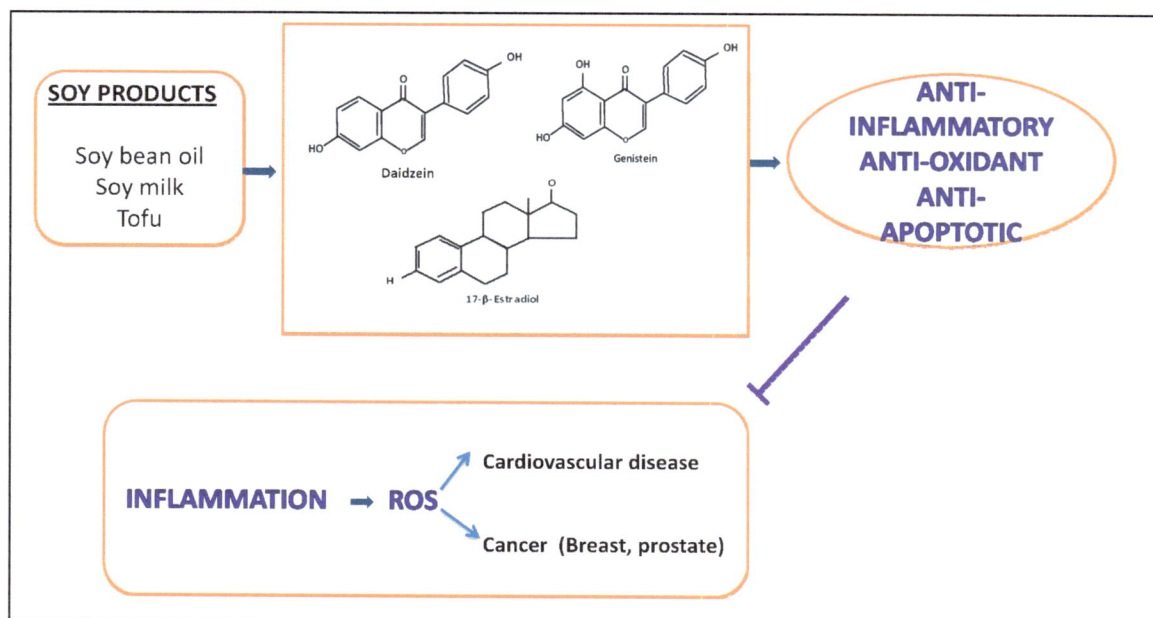

Figure 2: Beneficial effects of Soy proteins: Soy proteins are consumed in various forms. The major phytochemicals in soy are the isoflavones, genistein and daidzein. The beneficial effects of soy isoflavones are attributed to their similarity in structure to 17β-estradiol. Soy isoflavones are shown to have anti-inflammatory, anti-oxidant and anti-apoptotic properties.

Both in cell culture studies and *in vivo* in healthy males, genistein inhibited the activation of the redox-sensitive transcription factor, NFkB in prostate cancer cells and TNF-α induced NFkB activation [64]. Similarly, in primary and cancer lymphocytes, both genistein and daidzein decreased lipid peroxidation products and protected DNA from oxidative damage [65]. Soy supplement tablets (Novasoy-50 mg/day) taken by healthy men and women resulted in decreased oxidative stress markers [66]. Similarly soy supplements (100 mg/day Novasoy for 5 months) decreased serum prostate-specific antigen (PSA) levels compared to hormone therapy in patients with prostate cancer [67].

Genistein also protects animals against chemically induced mammary and prostate cancers [68]. *In vivo* studies with methylnitrosourea induced breast tumors in Sprague Dawley rats showed that genistein (20 mg/day) treated animals after 84 days had lowest number of palpable tumors compared to vehicle controls [69]. Gene expression profiling of prostate cells (LAPC-4) treated with genistein (1-30 μM) showed induction of antioxidant genes and metallothioneins that protect cells from ROS damage [70]. Daidzin (300 μM), a different isoflavone from soy, directly activated the catalase promoter and increased catalase mRNA expression in rat hepatoma H4IIE cells but the authors did not evaluate catalase enzyme activity [71].

The most recent study that re-affirmed the protective role of soy isoflavones in breast cancer patients came from the results of the Shanghai Breast cancer survival study, a large, population based cohort of 5042 female breast cancer survivors in China. This study concluded that there was a strong association between soy food intake and decreased mortality and recurrence of breast cancer [57] However, the American Cancer Society still cautions people to avoid concentrated soy extracts and consume only modest amount of soy containing foods. Therefore, more mechanistic studies are necessary to clarify the benefit/risk controversy associated with soy consumption and cancer prevention and treatment.

CONCLUSIONS

Though several natural products have tumor preventing activities, partially attributed to their ability to scavenge ROS production, more case-controlled studies are needed to confirm the beneficial anti-tumor effects of these compounds.

ACKNOWLEDGEMENTS

The authors wish to acknowledge the financial support of NIH grants RO1 HL074239 (NS), P20RR016477-09S2 (NS) and P20RR016477-09S4 (MAV).

REFERENCES

[1]   Petrelli NJ, Winer EP, Brahmer J, *et al.* Clinical Cancer Advances 2009: major research advances in cancer treatment, prevention, and screening--a report from the American Society of Clinical Oncology. J Clin Oncol 2009; 27(35): 6052-69.

[2]   Halliwell B. Oxidative stress and cancer: have we moved forward? Biochem J 2007; 401(1): 1-11.

[3]   Klaunig JE, Kamendulis LM. The role of oxidative stress in carcinogenesis. Annu Rev Pharmacol Toxicol 2004; 44: 239-67.

[4]   Circu ML, Aw TY. Reactive oxygen species, cellular redox systems, and apoptosis. Free Radic Biol Med 2010; 48(6): 749-62.

[5]   Forkink M, Smeitink JA, Brock R, Willems PH, Koopman WJ. Detection and manipulation of mitochondrial reactive oxygen species in mammalian cells. Biochim Biophys Acta 2010; 1797(6-7): 1034-44.

[6]   Kowaltowski AJ, de Souza-Pinto NC, Castilho RF, Vercesi AE. Mitochondria and reactive oxygen species. Free Radic Biol Med 2009; 47(4): 333-43.

[7]   Jaquet V, Scapozza L, Clark RA, Krause KH, Lambeth JD. Small-molecule NOX inhibitors: ROS-generating NADPH oxidases as therapeutic targets. Antioxid Redox Signal 2009; 11(10): 2535-52.

[8]   Cross JV, Templeton DJ. Regulation of signal transduction through protein cysteine oxidation. Antioxid Redox Signal 2006; 8(9-10): 1819-27.

[9]   Blokhina O, Virolainen E, Fagerstedt KV. Antioxidants, oxidative damage and oxygen deprivation stress: a review. Ann Bot 2003; 91 Spec No: 179-94.

[10]   Galecka E, Jacewicz R, Mrowicka M, Florkowski A, Galecki P. [Antioxidative enzymes--structure, properties, functions]. Pol Merkur Lekarski 2008; 25(147): 266-8.

[11]   Kalinina EV, Chernov NN, Saprin AN. Involvement of thio-, peroxi-, and glutaredoxins in cellular redox-dependent processes. Biochemistry (Mosc) 2008; 73(13): 1493-510.

[12]   Nguyen T, Nioi P, Pickett CB. The Nrf2-antioxidant response element signaling pathway and its activation by oxidative stress. J Biol Chem 2009; 284(20): 13291-5.

[13]   Zadak Z, Hyspler R, Ticha A, *et al.* Antioxidants and vitamins in clinical conditions. Physiol Res 2009; 58 Suppl 1: S13-7.

[14]   Iannitti T, Palmieri B. Antioxidant therapy effectiveness: an up to date. Eur Rev Med Pharmacol Sci 2009; 13(4): 245-78.

[15]   Balsano C, Alisi A. Antioxidant effects of natural bioactive compounds. Curr Pharm Des 2009; 15(26): 3063-73.

[16]   Weinberg F, Chandel NS. Reactive oxygen species-dependent signaling regulates cancer. Cell Mol Life Sci 2009; 66(23): 3663-73.

[17]   Zimmerman R, Cerutti P. Active oxygen acts as a promoter of transformation in mouse embryo C3H/10T1/2/C18 fibroblasts. Proc Natl Acad Sci U S A 1984; 81(7): 2085-7.

[18]   Szatrowski TP, Nathan CF. Production of large amounts of hydrogen peroxide by human tumor cells. Cancer Res 1991; 51(3): 794-8.

[19]   Guilford JM, Pezzuto JM. Natural products as inhibitors of carcinogenesis. Expert Opin Investig Drugs 2008; 17(9): 1341-52.

[20]   Nobili S, Lippi D, Witort E, *et al.* Natural compounds for cancer treatment and prevention. Pharmacol Res 2009; 59(6): 365-78.

[21]   Sarkar FH, Li Y, Wang Z, Kong D. Cellular signaling perturbation by natural products. Cell Signal 2009; 21(11): 1541-7.

[22]   Jurenka JS. Therapeutic applications of pomegranate (Punica granatum L.): a review. Altern Med Rev 2008; 13(2): 128-44.

[23]   Vieira O, Escargueil-Blanc I, Meilhac O, *et al.* Effect of dietary phenolic compounds on apoptosis of human cultured endothelial cells induced by oxidized LDL. Br J Pharmacol 1998; 123(3): 565-73.

[24]   Bell C, Hawthorne S. Ellagic acid, pomegranate and prostate cancer--a mini review. J Pharm Pharmacol 2008; 60(2): 139-44.

[25]   Pantuck AJ, Leppert JT, Zomorodian N, *et al.* Phase II study of pomegranate juice for men with rising prostate-specific antigen following surgery or radiation for prostate cancer. Clin Cancer Res 2006; 12(13): 4018-26.

[26]   Seeram NP, Aronson WJ, Zhang Y, *et al.* Pomegranate ellagitannin-derived metabolites inhibit prostate cancer growth and localize to the mouse prostate gland. J Agric Food Chem 2007; 55(19): 7732-7.

[27]   Tharappel JC, Lehmler HJ, Srinivasan C, *et al.* Effect of antioxidant phytochemicals on the hepatic tumor promoting activity of 3,3',4,4'-tetrachlorobiphenyl (PCB-77). Food Chem Toxicol 2008; 46(11): 3467-74.

[28]   Aiyer HS, Srinivasan C, Gupta RC. Dietary berries and ellagic acid diminish estrogen-mediated mammary tumorigenesis in ACI rats. Nutr Cancer 2008; 60(2): 227-34.

[29]   Gonzalez-Sarrias A, Espin JC, Tomas-Barberan FA, Garcia-Conesa MT. Gene expression, cell cycle arrest and MAPK signalling regulation in Caco-2 cells exposed to ellagic acid and its metabolites, urolithins. Mol Nutr Food Res 2009; 53(6): 686-98.

[30]   Narayanan BA, Narayanan NK, Stoner GD, Bullock BP. Interactive gene expression pattern in prostate cancer cells exposed to phenolic antioxidants. Life Sci 2002; 70(15): 1821-39.

[31]   Butt MS, Sultan MT. Green tea: nature's defense against malignancies. Crit Rev Food Sci Nutr 2009; 49(5): 463-73.

[32]   Pandey M, Gupta S. Green tea and prostate cancer: from bench to clinic. Front Biosci (Elite Ed) 2009; 1: 13-25.

[33]   McLarty J, Bigelow RL, Smith M, *et al.* Tea polyphenols decrease serum levels of prostate-specific antigen, hepatocyte growth factor, and vascular endothelial growth factor in prostate cancer patients and inhibit production of hepatocyte growth factor and vascular endothelial growth factor *in vitro*. Cancer Prev Res 2009; 2(7): 673-82.

[34]   Gupta S, Ahmad N, Nieminen AL, Mukhtar H. Growth inhibition, cell-cycle dysregulation, and induction of apoptosis by green tea constituent (-)-epigallocatechin-3-gallate in androgen-sensitive and androgen-insensitive human prostate carcinoma cells. Toxicol Appl Pharmacol 2000; 164(1): 82-90.

[35]   Gupta S, Hussain T, Mukhtar H. Molecular pathway for (-)-epigallocatechin-3-gallate-induced cell cycle arrest and apoptosis of human prostate carcinoma cells. Arch Biochem Biophys 2003; 410(1): 177-85.

[36]   Hastak K, Gupta S, Ahmad N, *et al.* Role of p53 and NF-kappaB in epigallocatechin-3-gallate-induced apoptosis of LNCaP cells. Oncogene 2003; 22(31): 4851-9.

[37]   Hussain T, Gupta S, Adhami VM, Mukhtar H. Green tea constituent epigallocatechin-3-gallate selectively inhibits COX-2 without affecting COX-1 expression in human prostate carcinoma cells. Int J Cancer 2005; 113(4): 660-9.

[38]   Kim MH, Chung J. Synergistic cell death by EGCG and ibuprofen in DU-145 prostate cancer cell line. Anticancer Res 2007; 27(6B): 3947-56.

[39]   Jagtap S, Meganathan K, Wagh V, *et al.* Chemoprotective mechanism of the natural compounds, epigallocatechin-3-O-gallate, quercetin and curcumin against cancer and cardiovascular diseases. Curr Med Chem 2009; 16(12): 1451-62.

[40]   Navarro-Peran E, Cabezas-Herrera J, Sanchez-Del-Campo L, Garcia-Canovas F, Rodriguez-Lopez JN. The anti-inflammatory and anti-cancer properties of epigallocatechin-3-gallate are mediated by folate cycle disruption, adenosine release and NF-kappaB suppression. Inflamm Res 2008; 57(10): 472-8.

[41]   Qanungo S, Das M, Haldar S, Basu A. Epigallocatechin-3-gallate induces mitochondrial membrane depolarization and caspase-dependent apoptosis in pancreatic cancer cells. Carcinogenesis 2005; 26(5): 958-67.

[42]   Lambert JD, Sang S, Yang CS. N-Acetylcysteine enhances the lung cancer inhibitory effect of epigallocatechin-3-gallate and forms a new adduct. Free Radic Biol Med 2008; 44(6): 1069-74.

[43]   Renaud S, de Lorgeril M. Wine, alcohol, platelets, and the French paradox for coronary heart disease. Lancet 1992; 339(8808):1523-6.

[44]   Brisdelli F, D'Andrea G, Bozzi A. Resveratrol: a natural polyphenol with multiple chemopreventive properties. Curr Drug Metab 2009; 10(6): 530-46.

[45]   Pervaiz S, Holme AL. Resveratrol: its biologic targets and functional activity. Antioxid Redox Signal 2009; 11(11): 2851-97.

[46]   Ulrich S, Wolter F, Stein JM. Molecular mechanisms of the chemopreventive effects of resveratrol and its analogs in carcinogenesis. Mol Nutr Food Res 2005; 49(5): 452-61.

[47]   Lee MH, Choi BY, Kundu JK, *et al.* Resveratrol suppresses growth of human ovarian cancer cells in culture and in a murine xenograft model: eukaryotic elongation factor 1A2 as a potential target. Cancer Res 2009; 69(18): 7449-58.

[48]   Opipari AW, Jr., Tan L, Boitano AE, *et al.* Resveratrol-induced autophagocytosis in ovarian cancer cells. Cancer Res 2004; 64(2): 696-703.

[49]   Jang M, Cai L, Udeani GO, *et al.* Cancer chemopreventive activity of resveratrol, a natural product derived from grapes. Science 1997; 275(5297): 218-20.

[50]   Miksits M, Wlcek K, Svoboda M, *et al.* Antitumor activity of resveratrol and its sulfated metabolites against human breast cancer cells. Planta Med 2009; 75(11): 1227-30.

[51]   Tang FY, Su YC, Chen NC, Hsieh HS, Chen KS. Resveratrol inhibits migration and invasion of human breast-cancer cells. Mol Nutr Food Res 2008; 52(6): 683-91.

[52]   Garvin S, Ollinger K, Dabrosin C. Resveratrol induces apoptosis and inhibits angiogenesis in human breast cancer xenografts *in vivo*. Cancer Lett 2006; 231(1): 113-22.

[53]   Olas B, Nowak P, Ponczek M, Wachowicz B. Resveratrol, a natural phenolic compound may reduce carbonylation proteins induced by peroxynitrite in blood platelets. Gen Physiol Biophys 2006; 25(2): 215-22.

[54]   Gresele P, Pignatelli P, Guglielmini G, *et al.* Resveratrol, at concentrations attainable with moderate wine consumption, stimulates human platelet nitric oxide production. J Nutr 2008; 138(9): 1602-8.

[55]   Robb EL, Page MM, Wiens BE, Stuart JA. Molecular mechanisms of oxidative stress resistance induced by resveratrol: Specific and progressive induction of MnSOD. Biochem Biophys Res Commun 2008; 367(2): 406-12.

[56]   Sareen D, Darjatmoko SR, Albert DM, Polans AS. Mitochondria, calcium, and calpain are key mediators of resveratrol-induced apoptosis in breast cancer. Mol Pharmacol 2007; 72(6): 1466-75.

[57]   Shu XO, Zheng Y, Cai H, *et al.* Soy food intake and breast cancer survival. Jama 2009; 302(22): 2437-43.

[58]   Cederroth CR, Nef S. Soy, phytoestrogens and metabolism: A review. Mol Cell Endocrinol 2009; 304(1-2): 30-42.

[59]   Messina M. Investigating the optimal soy protein and isoflavone intakes for women: a perspective. Womens Health (Lond Engl) 2008; 4(4): 337-56.

[60]   Murata M, Midorikawa K, Koh M, Umezawa K, Kawanishi S. Genistein and daidzein induce cell proliferation and their metabolites cause oxidative DNA damage in relation to isoflavone-induced cancer of estrogen-sensitive organs. Biochemistry 2004; 43(9): 2569-77.

[61]   Sonee M, Sum T, Wang C, Mukherjee SK. The soy isoflavone, genistein, protects human cortical neuronal cells from oxidative stress. Neurotoxicology 2004; 25(5): 885-91.

[62]   Sasaki M, Nakamura H, Tsuchiya S, *et al.* Quercetin-induced PC12 cell death accompanied by caspase-mediated DNA fragmentation. Biol Pharm Bull 2007; 30(4): 682-6.

[63]   Banerjee S, Li Y, Wang Z, Sarkar FH. Multi-targeted therapy of cancer by genistein. Cancer Lett 2008; 269(2): 226-42.

[64]   Davis JN, Kucuk O, Djuric Z, Sarkar FH. Soy isoflavone supplementation in healthy men prevents NF-kappa B activation by TNF-alpha in blood lymphocytes. Free Radic Biol Med 2001; 30(11): 1293-302.

[65]   Foti P, Erba D, Riso P, *et al.* Comparison between daidzein and genistein antioxidant activity in primary and cancer lymphocytes. Arch Biochem Biophys 2005; 433(2): 421-7.

[66]   Djuric Z, Chen G, Doerge DR, Heilbrun LK, Kucuk O. Effect of soy isoflavone supplementation on markers of oxidative stress in men and women. Cancer Lett 2001; 172(1): 1-6.

[67]   Hussain M, Banerjee M, Sarkar FH, *et al.* Soy isoflavones in the treatment of prostate cancer. Nutr Cancer 2003; 47(2): 111-7.

[68]   Pugalendhi P, Manoharan S, Panjamurthy K, Balakrishnan S, Nirmal MR. Antigenotoxic effect of genistein against 7,12-dimethylbenz[a]anthracene induced genotoxicity in bone marrow cells of female Wistar rats. Pharmacol Rep 2009; 61(2): 296-303.

[69]   Hooshmand S, Khalil DA, Murillo G, *et al.* The combination of genistin and ipriflavone prevents mammary tumorigenesis and modulates lipid profile. Clin Nutr 2008; 27(4): 643-8.

[70]   Raschke M, Rowland IR, Magee PJ, Pool-Zobel BL. Genistein protects prostate cells against hydrogen peroxide-induced DNA damage and induces expression of genes involved in the defence against oxidative stress. Carcinogenesis 2006; 27(11): 2322-30.

[71]   Rohrdanz E, Ohler S, Tran-Thi QH, Kahl R. The phytoestrogen daidzein affects the antioxidant enzyme system of rat hepatoma H4IIE cells. J Nutr 2002; 132(3): 370-5.

CHAPTER 8

Is there an Etiologic Role for Dietary Iron and Red Meat in Breast Cancer Development?

John Wilkinson IV[*]

Nutrition and Cancer Center, Department of Anatomy and Pathology, Joan C. Edwards School of Medicine, Marshall University, Huntington, WV, 25755, USA

Abstract: The purpose of this review is to examine the literature to determine what epidemiologic and experimental evidence exists that either supports or denies a role for iron in the etiology of breast cancer, paying particular attention to the dietary heme iron source of red meat. The importance of red meat as a dietary source of iron and the relationship between iron and oxidant stress are introduced. Epidemiologic and experimental studies of the relationship between iron and breast cancer are reviewed. Extant studies involving phase II detoxication gene interactions with red meat consumption and breast cancer or iron-related gene polymorphisms and breast cancer are also reviewed. In conclusion, a model by which red meat may impact breast cancer involving the delivery of dietary iron is proposed and discussed.

Keywords: Breast Cancer, Cancer, Diet, Epidemiology, Food, Gene Polymorphism, Glutathione, Heme, Iron, Meat, Menopause, Nutrition, Phase I Enzyme, Phase II Enzyme, Progesterone Receptor, Red Meat.

INTRODUCTION

The idea that specific dietary components have a meaningful impact on the risk for developing certain types of cancer, which implies that individuals have some degree of control over their risk, is of great lay and scientific interest. At the turn of the century, it seemed clear that diet was a significant factor within the broad spectrum of environmental influences that might impact the risk of developing certain cancers [1]. It was also clear that the role played by genetics in cancer susceptibility is to some extent influenced by diet and cooking practices. More than thirty large scale epidemiologic studies were underway, studies that might benefit from refinements possible due to the results of prior work, and their findings were greatly anticipated [2]. Research leading to the identification of individual components of natural dietary constituents with cancer preventive or therapeutic properties may form the basis of dietary supplement based chemopreventives [3-5]. Likewise, identification of dietary constituents that contribute to carcinogenic risk could provide a basis for modifying eating or perhaps food preparation behaviors to be less risky.

The purpose of this review is to examine the literature to determine what epidemiologic and experimental evidence exists that either supports or denies a role for iron and red meat consumption in the etiology of breast cancer. It is a caveat of such work that red meat may be a vector for the delivery of several "usual suspects", essentially becoming a surrogate for consumption of high fat, heterocyclic amines, and residual hormones, in addition to heme iron. It is also important to keep in mind that the impact of red meat may derive at least in part from how these individual components interact as opposed to how each of their individual impacts sum together. Nevertheless, in this review, particular attention (where possible) will be paid to the impact of heme iron within red meat's overall mechanism(s) of action. While we are evaluating studies that include total meat and processed meat, we are paying particular attention to red meat because the iron in heme is more readily absorbed than non-heme iron, [6, 7] and red meat is a high source of heme in the western diet [8].

---

*Address Correspondence to John Wilkinson IV: Nutrition and Cancer Center, Department of Anatomy and Pathology, Joan C. Edwards School of Medicine, Marshall University, Byrd Biotechnology Science Center, Room 336V, 1700 Third Avenue, Huntington WV, 25755, USA; E-mail: wilkinsonj@marshall.edu

Pier Paolo Claudio and Richard M. Niles (Eds)

Why is Dietary Iron a Suspect?

A recurrent theme concerning iron's mechanism of action involves the generation of oxidant stress by free iron, often iron derived by heme breakdown [9]. This is because, while iron is essential for the function of enzymes that participate in numerous critical cellular processes, including transit through the cell cycle, the reductive conversion of ribonucleotides to deoxyribonucleotides, electron transport, and others it nevertheless is a potent mediator of oxidative stress [10]. Iron donates electrons for the generation of the superoxide radical, and serves as both an electron donor and acceptor in the iron catalyzed Fenton reaction [11] [$H_2O_2 + Fe^{2+} \rightarrow Fe^{3+} + OH^- + OH^\bullet$] which generates hydroxyl radicals, and can also lead to the formation of ferryl radicals [12]. The toxicity and potential carcinogenicity of iron [13] is attributable in large part to its capacity to participate in the generation of such reactive species, which can directly damage cellular constituents, such as DNA, lipids and proteins [14-16]. Levels of antioxidant containing vegetables or vitamin supplements or the consumption of dietary fats may interact with this oxidant stress generation, rendering these as potentially confounding variables.

Has the Role of Dietary Iron in the Etiology of Breast Cancer been Directly Assessed?

Rodent studies indicate that low dietary iron intake, [17] or treatment with iron chelators [18-20] leads to inhibition of mammary cancer *in vivo*. Conversely, dietary iron supplementation has been shown to stimulate breast [17] and colon cancer [21-23]. The impact of iron intake as a specific nutritional factor affecting fibrocystic breast changes and breast cancer risk was evaluated in a case-control (346 fibrocystic cases, 248 breast cancer cases, 1040 controls) study of women in Shanghai, China [24]. Plasma ferritin levels were most significantly associated with development of fibrocystic disease (OR: 2.51, 95% CI: 1.16-5.45, p trend = 0.04). While dietary iron intake was not associated directly with an increased risk for breast cancer, nevertheless, among patients with non-proliferative fibrocystic changes, or all fibrocystic changes, high iron intake increased risk of breast cancer development significantly (OR: 2.63, 95% CI: 1.04-6.68, p = 0.02) (OR: 1.36, 95% CI: 0.74–2.49, p_{trend}=0.01) within these groups, respectively.

Serum or Tissue Iron Levels and Breast Cancer

Certain studies have attempted to identify interactions between tissue or serum iron biomarkers and breast cancer incidence; the varied results indicate a need for the development of validated biomarkers for whole body or systemic iron levels. In a case-control study, serum iron levels and malondialdehyde levels were higher in breast cancer patients than in controls, though the two measurements were not significantly correlated [25]. This occurred despite a lower reported (questionnaire based) intake of total and non-heme iron in the breast cancer group. Hair iron levels in breast cancer patients were found to be reduced in a case control study by Joo *et al.* [26] Toenail iron levels were not found to be associated with breast cancer status in a case-control study [27]. In a small case-control study in Taiwan, 13 elements, including iron, were measured in the serum from 25 patients with malignant breast cancer, 43 patients with benign breast cancer and 26 controls [28]. The serum level pattern of iron, cadmium and manganese were sufficient to discriminate between malignant disease and benign disease and controls. A nested case-control study wherein breast tissue zinc, iron, calcium, and selenium were evaluated found positive associations between tissue zinc, iron and calcium and breast cancer risk [29]. When menopausal status was taken into account, the iron association was only seen among post-menopausal women, and was very strong: OR, 2.77;95% CL, 1.25, 6.13; p_{trend}=0.008, while the zinc and calcium associations were not differentiated by menopausal status.

The potential role for iron in the etiology of breast cancer was the subject of a recent excellent review by Kabat and Rohan [30]. This article proposes a simple hypothesis that excess dietary iron will lead to extra free iron derived oxidant stress. The authors therefore discuss mechanisms of action for iron which involve oxidant stress generation, and subsequent cellular damage to lipids, hormones, DNA, as well as impact on wide ranging potential targets such as zinc-finger proteins. In a subsequent review Huang proposed complex mechanisms for iron's action involving menstruation's influence on iron availability leading to divergent changes in HIF1a protein activity and oxidant stress [31]. This has also been the subject of research from the Huang laboratory [32]. Given the existence of these two reviews which focus on iron and not on red meat consumption, this work will focus primarily on more recent developments and on red (and other) meats as dietary iron sources.

Epidemiologic Studies of Red Meat and Breast Cancer

Studies of red meat and breast cancer range widely in: 1) their specific dietary comparisons, 2) whether they discriminate between the menopausal status of cases and controls, 3) whether the clinical or biologic types of breast cancer are factored into the analysis, and 4) if the study is prospective or case-control. In addition, any specific cohort or population under study may also have geographical differences from other studies. This review considers any dietary comparisons that involve meat or meat types which contain a red meat category. The studies are next divided on the basis of menopausal status of the cases and controls.

Red Meat and Pre-Menopausal Breast Cancer

Roughly 25% of all breast cancer cases occur in Pre-menopausal women [33]. Premenopausal breast cancer is reported to be more clinically aggressive [34], which is consistent with a decreased survival relative to post-menopausal breast cancer. This is seen when comparing the 83% 5 year survival rate of women diagnosed with breast cancer before age 40 (which are likely to be predominantly pre-menopausal) with the 90% survival rate of women diagnosed after age 40, (4/5ths of whom can be considered post-menopausal) [35].

Epidemiologic reports of premenopausal breast cancer were recently reviewed in Taylor, Misra, and Mukherjee [36]. Their well-written meta-analyses reviewed the findings of 3 cohort and 7 case-control studies focused on the impact of red meat breast cancer development in pre-menopausal women. Their results indicates that high consumption of red meat imparts an increased risk in this group (summary relative risk 1.24 (95% CI; 1.08-1.42) heterogeneity test =0.005). While iron was part of their review of components within red meat that might contribute individually to the impact of red meat consumption, and the authors cite two articles [37, 38] that address the potential for iron to affect estrogen related cancer, the principal etiologic focus of their discussion was on heterocyclic amine production and on estrogen and progesterone receptor phenotypes [39, 40] and how these relate to breast cancer risk.

One study of note, the Nurses Health Study II, reported by Cho *et al.* stratified the cases by estrogen and progesterone receptor status (ER and PR), as an attempt at elucidating potential mechanisms through which red meat might influence cancer development [39]. In this large prospective study, 90, 659 pre-menopausal women were followed up for 12 years. Among ER+/PR+ cases, increasing intake of red meat increased risk of breast cancer development (OR for highest intake of more than 1.5 servings per day *vs.* 3 or fewer per week 1.97 (95% CI; 1.35-2.88; p^{trend} 0.001). A similar association with ER-/PR-cases was not seen.

Red Meat and Post-Menopausal Breast Cancer

Of the four studies that were found which analyze red meat or meat's impact on breast cancer specifically in post-menopausal populations, three support a role for red meat in the etiology of breast cancer. Red meat intake significantly increased breast cancer risk (p_{trend} =0.002) in a post-menopausal population in Washington State comprising 441 cases and 370 age matched controls [41]. In the UK Womens Cohort Study, dietary intake was assessed by questionnaire. The pre-menopausal findings of this study were reported in the previously cited review by Taylor *et al.* where High Total meat was found to confer higher risk for breast cancer among pre-menopausal women (OR=1.20, 95%CI: 0.86-1.68). Total, processed, and red meat consumption conferred even higher risk increases among post-menopausal women (OR for highest *vs.* lowest intake of red meat 1.56 (95%CI; 1.09-2.23) p^{trend} 0.040) [42]. A case-control study in Shanghai evaluated dietary intake of iron and fat in 1, 366 post-menopausal breast cancer cases and 1, 506 matched controls through validated questionnaires [43]. Results, adjusted for antioxidant, isoflavone and vitamin supplement intake, indicated dietary heme iron (animal source iron) intake was highly associated with breast cancer incidence (OR for highest *vs.* lowest quartile 1.56 [95% CI; 1.17-2.05, p^{trend} <0.01]) in post-menopausal women, despite a lack of association found with total dietary iron intake. Dietary fat intake interacted significantly with iron and was similarly associated with breast cancer, particularly in post-menopausal women. Interestingly, the intake of iron from vegetable sources was found to significantly decrease risk, until confounding variables such as antioxidant vitamin consumption were taken into account. In contrast to these other post-menopause specific studies, in the NIH-AARP Diet and Health Study, diets were assessed by baseline questionnaire and a meat cooking module in a large cohort of post-menopausal women. After 8 years of follow up, no association between red meat intake and increased breast cancer risk were found [44].

Red Meat and All Breast Cancer

In many studies, no distinction is made between pre-and post-menopausal cases and controls. As roughly 25% of breast cancer is pre-menopausal [33], it stands to reason that the remaining 75%, arguably the bulk of cases when all breast cancers are being evaluated, are post-menopausal. This implies that in these studies that post menopausal characteristics may have 3 times the influence of pre-menopausal disease on the outcomes of the analyses. This ratio may further increase as the mean age of the cohort increases.

In a meta-analysis of earlier studies, Missmer *et al.* [45] combined data from 8 North American and Western European prospective cohort studies of the impact of meat and dairy product consumption on breast cancer incidence in 2002. The pooled data indicated no risk derives from total, red or white meat consumption. In contrast, a report by Boyd *et al.* on dietary fat and breast cancer also included a meta-analysis of meat consumption (not red-meat) and breast cancer risk from 31 published studies [46]. The pooled findings indicated a summary relative risk for the highest partitioned group of meat consumption of 1.17 (95%CI : 1.06-1.29) for all studies, 1.13 (95% CI : 1.01-1.25) for twenty-two case-control studies, and 1.32 (95% CI : 1.12-1.56) for nine prospective studies. Thus, while certain past studies found no role for red meat as a risk factor for breast cancer, a very broad analysis [46] indicates high consumption of red meat is a significant risk factor. This current report will focus on studies that have reported data since these earlier analyses.

Four prospective and seven case control studies were found in which dietary consumption of red meat or iron were assessed for their association with breast cancer incidence, wherein findings were reported for "all women" regardless of menopausal status or where menopausal status was not taken into consideration. These studies are depicted in Fig. **1** using a forest plot to visually compare the studies using the parameters of number of cases (represented by square symbol outline size), hazard or odds ratio (depicted by the center of the square symbol) and the confidence intervals (extending to either side of the symbol). A dashed line running down the center of the plot indicates a ratio of 1, which would indicate no influence on incidence.

Five of these studies (two prospective, three case-control), along with another, which tested vegetables *vs.* "pork, potatoes and processed meat" did not find a positive association between red meat intake and breast cancer development. It should be noted that these include the two larger prospective studies of the four. In a case-control study of a population based in Heidelberg, Germany, the intake of many nutrients including β-carotene, copper, folate, raw vegetables, vitamin C and zinc were all associated with an inverse risk for breast cancer, while no association was found for dietary iron intake [47]. The DIETSCAN project examined three cohorts from the Netherlands, Sweden, and Italy to determine if particular dietary intake patterns corresponded to changes in breast cancer incidence [48]. Neither the high vegetable intake group (VEG) nor the high pork, processed meat and potatoes group (PPP) were found to be positively associated with breast cancer incidence, while a possible mild *protective* impact of the PPP pattern was seen for the Netherland cohort. The Center for Chronic Disease Prevention and Control in Canada released findings from a questionnaire based study of two years of pre study food habits for greater than 19, 000 cancer patients and 5000 controls drawn from eight provinces over the period of 1994 to 1997 [49]. While total and processed meat was found to be directly related to the risk of developing breast cancer, red meat consumption was not. A case-control study examining dietary intake and cooking preferences of specific meats found no important association between dietary red meat and breast cancer risk [50]. This group also stratified red meat results against NAT2 acetylator phenotype and PhIP (the heterocyclic amine, 2-amino-1-methyl-6-phenylimidazo[4, 5]pyridine) consumption to test for significant interactions, but found none.

The European Prospective Investigation into Cancer and Nutrition (EPIC) is a multi center study conducted in 23 centers across 10 European countries. In this study, dietary intake information was obtained using a validated questionnaire from a cohort of 319, 826 women recruited from 1992 through 1998 [51]. Within the 7119 breast cancer cases that developed during a median 8.8 years of follow up, red meat consumption was found to have no significant impact on breast cancer risk, despite a trend for high intakes of processed meat to slightly increase risk. In a later report from the EPIC study, the cohort had increased to 366, 521 women and 153, 457 men. While alcohol intake was strongly [52], and saturate fat weakly [53], associated with increases in breast cancer risk, again, no association was found with red meat intake [54]. Similarly, in a long term study of a Swedish cohort, the intake of total red meat, fresh red meat, or processed meat was found to have no impact on breast cancer risk [55]. It should be noted however that in the same study, an increased intake of pan fried meat was found to increase the risk for ER+/PR-tumors 1.45 fold (95% CI ; 1.03-2.03; P^{trend}=0.03).

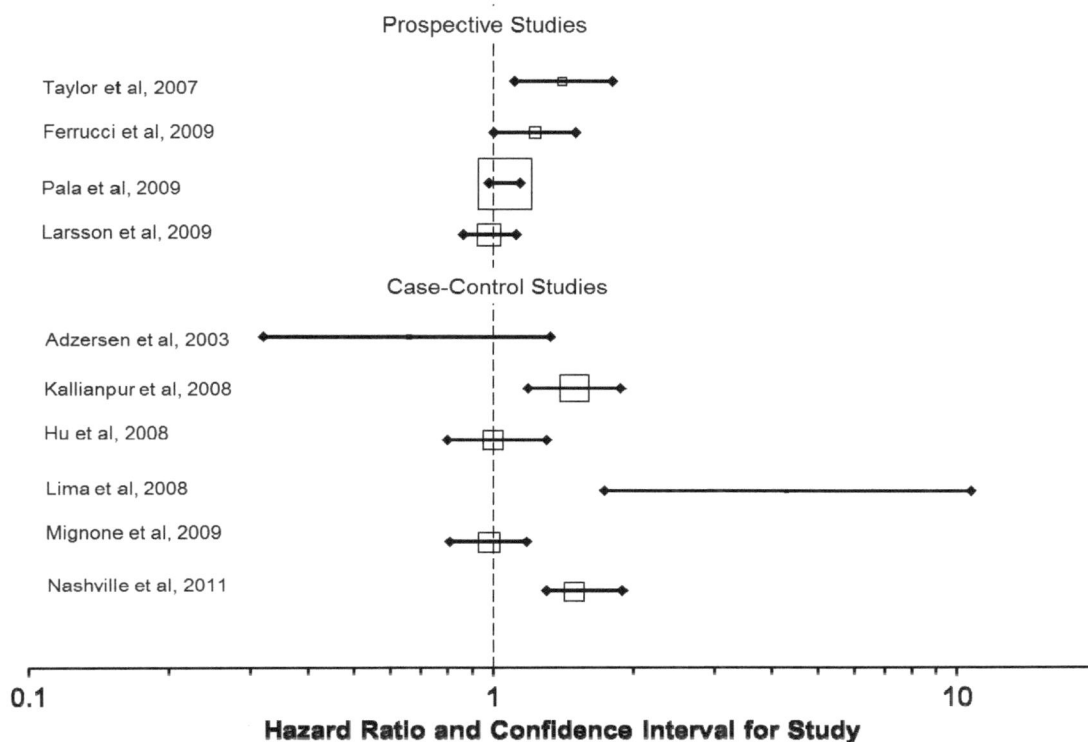

Figure 1: Forest Plot Depicting Studies of Breast Cancer Cohorts Where No Distinction Is Made Between Pre-And Post-Menopausal Women. The hazard or odds ratio (depicted by the center of the square symbols position on the x axis) and confidence intervals reported (extending to either side of the symbol) depict the relative risk of breast cancer incidence for the highest *vs.* the lowest quartile or quintile of red meat or iron intake. Included are all studies involving iron or red meat and breast cancer that have been published since the meta-analysis of Boyd [46]. Studies are divided by prospective and case-control designs. Author reference and year are depicted to the left of the hazard or odds ratio information. A dashed line running down the center of the plot indicates a ratio of 1, which would indicate no influence on incidence. The size of the square symbol outline represents the relative number of cases.

Five studies (two prospective and three case-control) indicated that high intake of either red meat or iron (along with another study that indicated a dietary pattern of "refined grain-meat-pickle") were associated with increased risk for breast cancer incidence. Findings from the UK Womens Cohort Study, adjusted for all women, indicate that high red meat consumption conferred significantly increased breast cancer incidence (OR for highest *vs.* lowest intake of red meat 1.41 (95% CI : 1.11-1.81) p^{trend} 0.007) [42]. Analysis of data from the US Prostate, Lung, Colorectal, and Ovarian Cancer Screening Trial revealed that dietary iron, processed and red meat were all associated with increased risk for development of breast cancer [56]. Interestingly, despite these associations, dietary iron was the only variable that showed a significant linear trend (OR for highest *vs.* lowest quintile 1.25 (95% CI; 1.02-1.52, p^{trend} <0.03)).

In the Shanghai Breast Cancer Study, animal source dietary iron (most likely heme iron) was found to be significantly associated with an increased risk for breast cancer in all women (OR 1.50; 95% CI (1.19-1.88) p^{trend} <0.01) [57]. When the dietary intake of various micronutrients among 89 breast cancer patients and 94 age matched controls was compared in Paraíba State, Brazil, consumption of red and fried meat was a strong risk factor (OR 4.30; (95% CI: 1.74-10.67), p_{trend} = 0.00) for breast cancer development [58]. Fruits, juices, beans and dairy products were protective. Analysis of a case control study based in Hong Kong, China with 438 breast cancer cases and 438 matched controls indicated dietary patterns that confer significant reductions and increases in risk [59]. While, after adjusting for confounding variables (age at menarche, live births, age at first live birth, months of breast feeding, BMI, history of benign breast disease, mother/sister/daughter with breast cancer, physical activity, passive smoking and total energy intake) high intake of the vegetable-fruit-soy-milk-poultry-fish pattern diet reduced risk (OR highest *vs.* lowest 0.26 (95% CI ; 0.17-0.42) p^{trend} <0.001), high intake of the refined grain-meat-pickle-pattern diet significantly increased risk (OR 2.58 (95% CI ; 1.53-4.34) p^{trend} <0.001). The Nashville Breast Health Study reported results taken from analysis of 2, 386 cases and 1, 703 controls from a population of women in Nashville, TN [60]. Dietary intake of red meat cooked by all methods was significantly associated with higher incidence of breast cancer (OR 1.5 (95% CI ; 1.2-1.8) p^{trend} <0.001). Stratification of the data indicated that the association was strongest for well done prepared red meat, and that meat derived mutagen intake was significantly associated in post-menopausal women only.

Phase I and Phase II Detoxication Enzymes, Red Meat, and Breast Cancer

Phase I and Phase II detoxication enzyme polymorphisms, as discussed by Reszka *et al.*, appear to interact with dietary factors, adjusting how the intake of red or processed meat affects an individual's risk for development of breast and other cancers [61]. Those studies which have attempted to identify specific polymorphic interactions between genes involved in phase I and phase II detoxication enzyme metabolism and dietary iron or red meat consumption and how these may impact breast cancer risk are reported in this section. There are three reports involving the sulfotransferase 1A1 gene and the n-acetyltransferase 1 and 2 genes.

Results from a small case control study of an Iowa cohort of postmenopausal women probed by questionnaire (156 cases, 332 controls) revealed an intriguing relationship between phase I metabolism and the risk for breast cancer development imparted by red meat [62]. Individuals carrying the (arg)213(his) allele of the sulfotransferase 1A1 gene were found to be at significantly increased risk for breast cancer development (his frequency was 41.6% in cases *vs.* 34.1% in controls, p=0.03). This risk increased as the number of his alleles increased (his/his homozygotes had an 80% increase in risk, 95%CI 1.0-3.2;p=0.04). Interestingly, increasing "doneness" of red meat intake increased the risk of breast cancer in women with the wild type alleles (arg/arg; p_{trend}=0.01), had a lesser impact on women heterozygous carriers of the his allele (arg/his; p_{trend}=0.10), and had no impact on homozygous his carriers (his/his). These results implicate the action of sulfotransferase 1A1 in the production of red meat derived factors that contribute to the development of breast cancer, in post-menopausal women.

Results from a small case-control study in the Netherlands (229 cases, 264 controls) indicated that red meat consumption was not a significant risk factor for breast cancer development, even when stratified across NAT1 and NAT2 or GSTM1 carrier *vs.* null phenotypes [63]. In contrast, the later Danish "Diet, Cancer and Health" cohort study found that the impact of red meat consumption as a risk factor for breast cancer development may depend on the N-acetyl transferase (NAT) 1 and 2 phenotypes [64]. Total, red, and processed meat consumption increased risk respectively by 1.09 (95% CI, 1.02-1.17), 1.15 (95% CI, 1.01-1.31) and 1.23 (95% CI, 1.04-1.45) fold per 25g of daily intake. The interaction between this increased risk and NAT phenotype indicate that increased risk is associated with the intermediate/fast NAT2 acetylator phenotype. This may provide insight into studies wherein meat intake does not appear to enhance risk – some populations may be enriched with individuals genetically more susceptible to the influence of dietary meat intake.

Iron Gene Polymorphisms and Breast Cancer

Certain studies have attempted to identify interactions between polymorphisms in genes involved in iron homeostasis and breast cancer incidence. Two have found associations with breast cancer incidence while two have not. A study of C282Y allele frequency of the hemochromatosis associated HFE gene in a Tennessee breast cancer patient population revealed a significant increase over various control groups, and an overall increased risk based on C282Y allele dosage (p trend = 0.01) [65]. In a Turkish case-control study, the incidence of the H63D polymorphism of the HFE gene was determined (no C282Y polymorphisms were present) and compared between patient and control groups [66]. The incidence of H63D in cancer patients (22.2%) was nearly twice that among controls (14%); statistical analysis determined that the H63D polymorphism increased risk for breast cancer approximately two fold.

Various polymorphisms within four iron related genes (HFE, TFR1, TFR2, and FPN) were compared between breast cancer patients and controls in a German population based case-control study [67]. No associations were discovered within this population. In a Finnish case-control study of male breast cancer, the H63D and C282Y variants of the HFE gene were found to have no association with disease; rather they were associated with carriers of a common BRCA2 mutation (9346(-2)A→G) [68].

SUMMARY

To answer the question offered by the title of this review, it is expedient to focus the inquiry into two simpler questions: Are dietary iron and red meat risk factors for breast cancer for the general population, and are they risk factors for subsets of the population? The conclusions we can draw from the epidemiologic work reviewed herein can be summarized as: 1) the influence of red meat and iron on the development of all breast cancers in large populations (if any) can be difficult to discern; and 2) in smaller subsets of the broad population or of breast cancer cases the influence of red meat and iron on incidence is more readily revealed. For example, when studies of pre-menopausal breast cancer are focused on, Taylor *et al.* report a summary relative risk for high red meat consumption of 1.24 ((95% CI; 1.08-1.42) heterogeneity test =0.005) [69]. One specific study within their analysis, the Nurses Health Study II, reported that red meat derived risk was more significant for ER+/PR+ cases, a further subset within pre-menopausal cancer [70].

The role of iron may also be more readily discernable upon stratifying the data to seek interactions with genetic factors within the population under study. For example, epidermal growth factor receptor gene simple sequence CA repeat polymorphisms may interact with dietary factors such as red meat intake to affect risk of breast cancer development [71]. Among 616 cases and 1072 controls, the group of women with two long alleles were more strongly influenced by diet: high red meat intake increased risk more than ten-fold (OR 10.68; 95%CI, 1.57-72.58), while high vegetable intake was most protective (OR 0.07; 95%CI, 0.004-1.07) in this group. In another example, in post-menopausal women from the American Cancer Society Prevention II Nutrition Cohort, dietary iron intake and polymorphisms of four genes involved in oxidant stress detoxication were evaluated to determine their potential role in breast cancer development [72]. A dose trend for total number of "risk alleles" associated with increased breast cancer incidence was identified (P<0.04), with women carrying three or more risk alleles having a 1.56 fold increased risk for breast cancer. Dietary iron and iron supplement intake interacted significantly with genetic status, with women in the highest iron intake quartile (or who used iron supplements) who also carry three or more risk alleles having more than a two fold increased risk for breast cancer.

There were few specific studies of post-menopausal cancer, possibly as studies that do not differentiate between menopausal status nevertheless derive their findings principally from post-menopausal disease, as this constitutes roughly 75% of breast cancers. Of the four studies reviewed herein, in one case-control and one prospective, red meat was reported to significantly increase the risk for breast cancer, in another large case-control study (3, 452 cases, 3, 474 controls) animal source iron (compared to vegetable source iron) was found to be a significant risk factor, while in the final prospective study, no association was found between red meat consumption and iron.

The bulk of the studies under review however do not differentiate breast cancers across menopausal status for the cases. Boyd's meta-analysis reveals an overall trend for meat to confer increased hazard of developing breast cancer (1.17 (95% CI : 1.06-1.29) for all studies) [46]. Of the subsequent studies reported herein, some indicated no association between red meat consumption and breast cancer (these included the EPIC and other large prospective studies), while a few reported significant increases in risk associated with high consumption of red meat, total or processed or fried meat, dietary patterns that include meat, or dietary iron (see Fig. **1**). Given that the findings of more recent studies are not uniformly negative (split with 5 finding associated risk, 5 not), and the strength of the prior 31 study meta-analysis of Boyd *et al.*, it seems clear that under some circumstances, in certain populations, meat or red meat consumption contributes to breast cancer development. The development of an iron biomarker that would permit the establishment of dietary iron intake independent of diet recall would greatly facilitate the elucidation of irons role in the etiology of breast cancer (and other chronic diseases).

Huang's Hypothesis

Iron's influence on the development of breast cancer may ultimately be understood in simple terms where increased iron intake correlates with greater oxidant stress production and more cellular damage leading to accelerated progression, as proposed by Kabat and Rohan [30]. Huang proposes that an elegant dichotomous relationship exists between iron and breast cancer that is dependent upon menopausal status [31]. In pre-menopausal women, a relative state of anemia caused by menstruation leads to increased activity of HIF1α, increased angiogenesis, and ultimately more recurrence of breast cancer. In post-menopausal women, the increased iron arising from abrogation of menstrual loss, leads to increased oxidant stress and drives progression of the disease. This hypothesis thus includes the general mechanism proposed by Kabat and Rohan, but also attempts to explain the more aggressive disease seen in premenopausal women.

The implications of this hypothesis regarding the role of iron derived from dietary sources such as red meat are worth discussion. Essentially, Huang's proposal introduces us to the concept that, while oxidant stress which can derive from iron excess plays a negative or damaging (or progressive in cancer terms) role is a generally well accepted precept, a lack of iron may also influence events (such as angiogenesis) that drive progression. Thus, while dietary iron excess may drive progression through oxidant stress related damage, it also may attenuate the ability of cells to stimulate angiogenesis by providing a sufficiency of iron to permit HIF1α degradation. Certain recent experimental work supports this hypothesis, wherein iron deficiency leads to enhanced tumorigenesis in animal models [32]. Given the findings of Taylor *et al.*'s meta-analysis of pre-menopausal cancer, which reports a summary relative risk for high red meat consumption of 1.24 ((95% CI ; 1.08-1.42) heterogeneity test =0.005), it would seem that the increased risk due to high dietary iron intake may still take place in the context of menstruation [69]. This could be because oxidant stress is a stronger effect than that derived from HIF1α activity, or may indicate that the two processes, despite being dependent on different iron conditions, may combine their influences. For instance, menstruating women in the highest quartile of dietary iron intake may be subjected to periodic conditions of high iron, yielding increases in oxidant stress and periodic iron deficiency, and subsequent bursts of HIF1α activity. Of course, the pleiotropic nature of red meat consumption, which is delivering other constituents (in addition to iron) with potential to impact progression, could also help to explain the findings.

Perhaps these competing events that may derive from the extremes of iron intake, each of which may directly influence breast cancer progression, make it more difficult to discern epidemiologic relationships between dietary iron intake and disease incidence, as these are usually evaluated for significance *via* a linear trend model. From a health perspective, should Huang's hypothesis be supported, the question that springs to mind is whether a cellular concentration range exists where HIF1α degradation is not impaired due to lack of iron and oxidant stress generation is not greatly enhanced due to its relative abundance. Further, how readily can dietary practices achieve such a balance? Huang's hypothesis [31] clearly indicates there are dangers inherent to either extreme.

Future studies would benefit from a valid biomarker for iron consumption, eliminating the possibility of recall bias due to reliance on questionnaire-derived data. In addition, genetic polymorphic profile of genes involved in breast cancer biology, cellular and systemic iron homeostasis, and detoxication enzymes will undoubtedly permit the identification of subsets of the population at high risk for breast cancer development when challenged with high dietary iron intake. Identifying the specific polymorphisms and genes to test should be a high priority in preparation for future epidemiologic studies.

ACKNOWLEDGEMENTS

The author wishes to acknowledge the support of the NIH NCI (1R21CA133701) during the preparation of this review.

REFERENCES

[1] Willett WC. Diet and cancer. Oncologist 2000; 5(5): 393-404.

[2] Willett WC. Diet and cancer: one view at the start of the millennium. Cancer Epidemiol Biomarkers Prev 2001; 10(1): 3-8.

[3] Wilkinson J,IV, Clapper ML. Detoxication enzymes and chemoprevention. Proc Soc Exp Biol Med 1997; 216(2): 192-200.

[4] Wilkinson J,IV, Pietsch EC, Torti SV, Torti FM. Ferritin regulation by oxidants and chemopreventive xenobiotics. Adv Enzyme Regul 2003; 43: 135-51.

[5] Jiao Y, Wilkinson J,IV, Di X, Wang W, Hatcher H, Kock ND, *et al.* Curcumin, a cancer chemopreventive and chemotherapeutic agent, is a biologically active iron chelator. Blood 2009; 113(2): 462-9.

[6] Bjorn-Rasmussen E, Hallberg L, Isaksson B, Arvidsson B. Food iron absorption in man. Applications of the two-pool extrinsic tag method to measure heme and nonheme iron absorption from the whole diet. J Clin Invest 1974; 53(1): 247-55.

[7] Hallberg L, Bjorn-Rasmussen E, Howard L, Rossander L. Dietary heme iron absorption. A discussion of possible mechanisms for the absorption-promoting effect of meat and for the regulation of iron absorption. Scand J Gastroenterol 1979; 14(7): 769-79.

[8] Takkunen H, Seppanen R. Iron deficiency and dietary factors in Finland. Am J Clin Nutr 1975; 28(10): 1141-7.

[9] Tappel A. Heme of consumed red meat can act as a catalyst of oxidative damage and could initiate colon, breast and prostate cancers, heart disease and other diseases. Med Hypotheses 2007; 68(3): 562-4.

[10] Bae YJ, Yeon JY, Sung CJ, Kim HS, Sung MK. Dietary intake and serum levels of iron in relation to oxidative stress in breast cancer patients. J Clin Biochem Nutr 2009; 45(3): 355-60.

[11] Fenton HJH. Oxidation of tartaric acid in presence of iron. J Chem Soc 1894; 65: 899-910.

[12] Henle ES, Linn S. Formation, prevention, and repair of DNA damage by iron/hydrogen peroxide. The Journal of biological chemistry 1997; 272(31): 19095-8.

[13] Toyokuni S. Role of iron in carcinogenesis: cancer as a ferrotoxic disease. Cancer Sci 2009; 100(1): 9-16.

[14] Boutin AC, Shirali P, Garcon G, Gosset P, Leleu B, Marez T, *et al.* Peripheral markers (Clara cell protein and alpha-glutathione S-transferase) and lipidoperoxidation (malondialdehyde) assessment in Sprague-Dawley rats instilled with haematite and benzo[a]pyrene. J Appl Toxicol 1998; 18(1): 39-45.

[15] Garry S, Nesslany F, Aliouat E, Haguenoer JM, Marzin D. Hematite (Fe(2)O(3)) enhances benzo[a]pyrene genotoxicity in endotracheally treated rat, as determined by Comet Assay. Mutat Res 2003; 538(1-2): 19-29.

[16] Garry S, Nesslany F, Aliouat el M, Haguenoer JM, Marzin D. Potent genotoxic activity of benzo[a]pyrene coated onto hematite measured by unscheduled DNA synthesis *in vivo* in the rat. Mutagenesis 2003; 18(5): 449-55.

[17] Thompson HJ, Kennedy K, Witt M, Juzefyk J. Effect of dietary iron deficiency or excess on the induction of mammary carcinogenesis by 1-methyl-1-nitrosourea. Carcinogenesis 1991; 12(1): 111-4.

[18] Wang F, Elliott RL, Head JF. Inhibitory effect of deferoxamine mesylate and low iron diet on the 13762NF rat mammary adenocarcinoma. Anticancer Res 1999; 19(1A): 445-50.

[19] Jiang XP, Wang F, Yang DC, Elliott RL, Head JF. Induction of apoptosis by iron depletion in the human breast cancer MCF-7 cell line and the 13762NF rat mammary adenocarcinoma *in vivo*. Anticancer Res 2002; 22(5): 2685-92.

[20] Hoke EM, Maylock CA, Shacter E. Desferal inhibits breast tumor growth and does not interfere with the tumoricidal activity of doxorubicin. Free Radic Biol Med 2005; 39(3): 403-11.

[21] Sesink AL, Termont DS, Kleibeuker JH, Van der Meer R. Red meat and colon cancer: the cytotoxic and hyperproliferative effects of dietary heme. Cancer Res 1999; 59(22): 5704-9.

[22] Pierre F, Tache S, Petit CR, Van der Meer R, Corpet DE. Meat and cancer: haemoglobin and haemin in a low-calcium diet promote colorectal carcinogenesis at the aberrant crypt stage in rats. Carcinogenesis 2003; 24(10): 1683-90.

[23] Bastide NM, Pierre FH, Corpet DE. Heme iron from meat and risk of colorectal cancer: a meta-analysis and a review of the mechanisms involved. Cancer Prev Res (Phila) 2011; 4(2): 177-84.

[24]   Moore AB, Shannon J, Chen C, Lampe JW, Ray RM, Lewis SK, *et al*. Dietary and stored iron as predictors of breast cancer risk: A nested case-control study in Shanghai. Int J Cancer 2009; 125(5): 1110-7.

[25]   Bae YJ, Yeon JY, Sung CJ, Kim HS, Sung MK. Dietary intake and serum levels of iron in relation to oxidative stress in breast cancer patients. J Clin Biochem Nutr 2009; 45(3): 355-60.

[26]   Joo NS, Kim SM, Jung YS, Kim KM. Hair iron and other minerals' level in breast cancer patients. Biol Trace Elem Res 2009; 129(1-3): 28-35.

[27]   Garland M, Morris JS, Colditz GA, Stampfer MJ, Spate VL, Baskett CK, *et al*. Toenail trace element levels and breast cancer: a prospective study. Am J Epidemiol 1996; 144(7): 653-60.

[28]   Wu HD, Chou SY, Chen DR, Kuo HW. Differentiation of serum levels of trace elements in normal and malignant breast patients. Biol Trace Elem Res 2006; 113(1): 9-18.

[29]   Cui Y, Vogt S, Olson N, Glass AG, Rohan TE. Levels of zinc, selenium, calcium, and iron in benign breast tissue and risk of subsequent breast cancer. Cancer Epidemiol Biomarkers Prev 2007; 16(8): 1682-5.

[30]   Kabat GC, Rohan TE. Does excess iron play a role in breast carcinogenesis? An unresolved hypothesis. Cancer Causes Control 2007; 18(10): 1047-53.

[31]   Huang X. Does iron have a role in breast cancer? Lancet Oncol 2008; 9(8): 803-7.

[32]   Jian J, Yang Q, Dai J, Eckard J, Axelrod D, Smith J, *et al*. Effects of iron deficiency and iron overload on angiogenesis and oxidative stress-a potential dual role for iron in breast cancer. Free Radic Biol Med 2011; 50(7): 841-7.

[33]   Theriault RL, Sellin RV. Estrogen-replacement therapy in younger women with breast cancer. J Natl Cancer Inst Monogr 1994; (16): 149-52.

[34]   Anders CK, Hsu DS, Broadwater G, Acharya CR, Foekens JA, Zhang Y, *et al*. Young age at diagnosis correlates with worse prognosis and defines a subset of breast cancers with shared patterns of gene expression. J Clin Oncol 2008; 26(20): 3324-30.

[35]   ACS ACS. Breast Cancer Facts and Figures 2009-2010 Atlanta: American Cancer Society, Inc.

[36]   Taylor VH, Misra M, Mukherjee SD. Is red meat intake a risk factor for breast cancer among premenopausal women? Breast Cancer Res Treat 2009; 117(1): 1-8.

[37]   Wyllie S, Liehr JG. Enhancement of estrogen-induced renal tumorigenesis in hamsters by dietary iron. Carcinogenesis 1998; 19(7): 1285-90.

[38]   Liehr JG, Jones JS. Role of iron in estrogen-induced cancer. Curr Med Chem 2001; 8(7): 839-49.

[39]   Cho E, Chen WY, Hunter DJ, Stampfer MJ, Colditz GA, Hankinson SE, *et al*. Red meat intake and risk of breast cancer among premenopausal women. Arch Intern Med 2006; 166(20): 2253-9.

[40]   Linos E, Willett WC, Cho E, Colditz G, Frazier LA. Red meat consumption during adolescence among premenopausal women and risk of breast cancer. Cancer Epidemiol Biomarkers Prev 2008; 17(8): 2146-51.

[41]   Shannon J, Cook LS, Stanford JL. Dietary intake and risk of postmenopausal breast cancer (United States). Cancer Causes Control 2003; 14(1): 19-27.

[42]   Taylor EF, Burley VJ, Greenwood DC, Cade JE. Meat consumption and risk of breast cancer in the UK Women's Cohort Study. Br J Cancer 2007; 96(7): 1139-46.

[43]   Kallianpur AR, Lee SA, Gao YT, Lu W, Zheng Y, Ruan ZX, *et al*. Dietary animal-derived iron and fat intake and breast cancer risk in the Shanghai Breast Cancer Study. Breast Cancer Res Treat 2008; 107(1): 123-32.

[44]   Kabat GC, Cross AJ, Park Y, Schatzkin A, Hollenbeck AR, Rohan TE, *et al*. Meat intake and meat preparation in relation to risk of postmenopausal breast cancer in the NIH-AARP diet and health study. Int J Cancer 2009; 124(10): 2430-5.

[45]   Missmer SA, Smith-Warner SA, Spiegelman D, Yaun SS, Adami HO, Beeson WL, *et al*. Meat and dairy food consumption and breast cancer: a pooled analysis of cohort studies. Int J Epidemiol 2002; 31(1): 78-85.

[46]   Boyd NF, Stone J, Vogt KN, Connelly BS, Martin LJ, Minkin S. Dietary fat and breast cancer risk revisited: a meta-analysis of the published literature. Br J Cancer 2003; 89(9): 1672-85.

[47]   Adzersen KH, Jess P, Freivogel KW, Gerhard I, Bastert G. Raw and cooked vegetables, fruits, selected micronutrients, and breast cancer risk: a case-control study in Germany. Nutr Cancer 2003; 46(2): 131-7.

[48]   Mannisto S, Dixon LB, Balder HF, Virtanen MJ, Krogh V, Khani BR, *et al*. Dietary patterns and breast cancer risk: results from three cohort studies in the DIETSCAN project. Cancer Causes Control 2005; 16(6): 725-33.

[49]   Hu J, La Vecchia C, DesMeules M, Negri E, Mery L. Meat and fish consumption and cancer in Canada. Nutr Cancer 2008; 60(3): 313-24.

[50]   Mignone LI, Giovannucci E, Newcomb PA, Titus-Ernstoff L, Trentham-Dietz A, Hampton JM, *et al*. Meat consumption, heterocyclic amines, NAT2, and the risk of breast cancer. Nutr Cancer 2009; 61(1): 36-46.

[51]   Pala V, Krogh V, Berrino F, Sieri S, Grioni S, Tjonneland A, *et al.* Meat, eggs, dairy products, and risk of breast cancer in the European Prospective Investigation into Cancer and Nutrition (EPIC) cohort. Am J Clin Nutr 2009; 90(3): 602-12.

[52]   Sieri S, Krogh V, Ferrari P, Berrino F, Pala V, Thiebaut AC, *et al.* Dietary fat and breast cancer risk in the European Prospective Investigation into Cancer and Nutrition. Am J Clin Nutr 2008; 88(5): 1304-12.

[53]   Tjonneland A, Christensen J, Olsen A, Stripp C, Thomsen BL, Overvad K, *et al.* Alcohol intake and breast cancer risk: the European Prospective Investigation into Cancer and Nutrition (EPIC). Cancer Causes Control 2007; 18(4): 361-73.

[54]   Gonzalez CA, Riboli E. Diet and cancer prevention: Contributions from the European Prospective Investigation into Cancer and Nutrition (EPIC) study. Eur J Cancer 2010; 46(14): 2555-62.

[55]   Larsson SC, Bergkvist L, Wolk A. Long-term meat intake and risk of breast cancer by oestrogen and progesterone receptor status in a cohort of Swedish women. Eur J Cancer 2009; 45(17): 3042-6.

[56]   Ferrucci LM, Cross AJ, Graubard BI, Brinton LA, McCarty CA, Ziegler RG, *et al.* Intake of meat, meat mutagens, and iron and the risk of breast cancer in the Prostate, Lung, Colorectal, and Ovarian Cancer Screening Trial. Br J Cancer 2009; 101(1): 178-84.

[57]   Kallianpur AR, Lee SA, Gao YT, Lu W, Zheng Y, Ruan ZX, *et al.* Dietary animal-derived iron and fat intake and breast cancer risk in the Shanghai Breast Cancer Study. Breast Cancer Res Treat 2008; 107(1): 123-32.

[58]   Lima FE, Latorre Mdo R, Costa MJ, Fisberg RM. Diet and cancer in Northeast Brazil: evaluation of eating habits and food group consumption in relation to breast cancer. Cad Saude Publica 2008; 24(4): 820-8.

[59]   Zhang CX, Ho SC, Fu JH, Cheng SZ, Chen YM, Lin FY. Dietary patterns and breast cancer risk among Chinese women. Cancer Causes Control 2011; 22(1): 115-24.

[60]   Fu Z, Deming SL, Fair AM, Shrubsole MJ, Wujcik DM, Shu X, *et al.*, editors. Well-done meat intake and meat-derived mutagen exposures in relation to breast cancer risk: The Nashville Breast Health Study. American Association For Cancer Research 2011 Annual Meeting; 2011 April; Orlando FL.

[61]   Reszka E, Wasowicz W, Gromadzinska J. Genetic polymorphism of xenobiotic metabolising enzymes, diet and cancer susceptibility. Br J Nutr 2006; 96(4): 609-19.

[62]   Zheng W, Xie D, Cerhan JR, Sellers TA, Wen W, Folsom AR. Sulfotransferase 1A1 polymorphism, endogenous estrogen exposure, well-done meat intake, and breast cancer risk. Cancer Epidemiol Biomarkers Prev 2001; 10(2): 89-94.

[63]   van der Hel OL, Peeters PH, Hein DW, Doll MA, Grobbee DE, Ocke M, *et al.* GSTM1 null genotype, red meat consumption and breast cancer risk (The Netherlands). Cancer Causes Control 2004; 15(3): 295-303.

[64]   Egeberg R, Olsen A, Autrup H, Christensen J, Stripp C, Tetens I, *et al.* Meat consumption, N-acetyl transferase 1 and 2 polymorphism and risk of breast cancer in Danish postmenopausal women. Eur J Cancer Prev 2008;17(1): 39-47.

[65]   Kallianpur AR, Hall LD, Yadav M, Christman BW, Dittus RS, Haines JL, *et al.* Increased prevalence of the HFE C282Y hemochromatosis allele in women with breast cancer. Cancer Epidemiol Biomarkers Prev 2004; 13(2): 205-12.

[66]   Gunel-Ozcan A, Alyilmaz-Bekmez S, Guler EN, Guc D. HFE H63D mutation frequency shows an increase in Turkish women with breast cancer. BMC Cancer 2006; 6: 37.

[67]   Abraham BK, Justenhoven C, Pesch B, Harth V, Weirich G, Baisch C, *et al.* Investigation of genetic variants of genes of the hemochromatosis pathway and their role in breast cancer. Cancer Epidemiol Biomarkers Prev 2005; 14(5): 1102-7.

[68]   Syrjakoski K, Fredriksson H, Ikonen T, Kuukasjarvi T, Autio V, Matikainen MP, *et al.* Hemochromatosis gene mutations among Finnish male breast and prostate cancer patients. Int J Cancer 2006; 118(2): 518-20.

[69]   Taylor VH, Misra M, Mukherjee SD. Is red meat intake a risk factor for breast cancer among premenopausal women? Breast Cancer Res Treat 2009; 117(1): 1-8.

[70]   Cho E, Spiegelman D, Hunter DJ, Chen WY, Stampfer MJ, Colditz GA, *et al.* Premenopausal fat intake and risk of breast cancer. J Natl Cancer Inst 2003; 95(14): 1079-85.

[71]   Brandt B, Hermann S, Straif K, Tidow N, Buerger H, Chang-Claude J. Modification of breast cancer risk in young women by a polymorphic sequence in the egfr gene. Cancer Res 2004; 64(1): 7-12.

[72]   Hong CC, Ambrosone CB, Ahn J, Choi JY, McCullough ML, Stevens VL, *et al.* Genetic variability in iron-related oxidative stress pathways (Nrf2, NQ01, NOS3, and HO-1), iron intake, and risk of postmenopausal breast cancer. Cancer Epidemiol Biomarkers Prev 2007; 16(9): 1784-94.

CHAPTER 9

Isothiocyanates Target Carcinogenesis During Tumor Initiation, Promotion and Progression

Mary Allison Wolf and Pier Paolo Claudio[*]

Nutrition and Cancer Center, Departments of Biochemistry and Microbiology, Joan C. Edwards School of Medicine, Marshall University, Huntington, WV, USA

Abstract: Isothiocyanates (ITCs) are phytochemicals produced from the hydrolysis of glucosinolates, which are found at high concentrations in cruciferous vegetables. Vegetables of the Cruciferae family include, among others, broccoli, cauliflower, gardencress, watercress, and cabbage. A number of studies using animal models have suggested that certain ITCs are capable of preventing breast, lung, and prostate carcinogenesis. Additionally, certain ITCs such as sulforaphane (SFN), benzyl (BITC), and phenethyl (PEITC) isothiocyanate have been shown to elicit strong chemotherapeutic properties. SFN, BITC, and PEITC are suggested to target several cellular pathways that inhibit growth, induce apoptosis, and prevent migration, and are presently being investigated for their therapeutic potential. Work on ITCs is progressing quickly from bench to beside, and currently there are several ongoing clinical trials. One study is investigating PEITC's ability to inhibit lung carcinogenesis, while another trial is investigating how PEITC affects lymphoproliferative disorders, specifically in patients who have received the chemotherapeutic drug, fludarabine. Additionally, a Phase II clinical trial is investigating whether SFN can modulate the level of prostate specific antigen in patients with recurrent prostate cancer. This chapter will give an overview of the previously mentioned ITCs, and their reported ability to inhibit carcinogenesis *in vivo* and *in vitro* at three stages: initiation, promotion, and progression.

Keywords: Angiogenesis, Apoptosis, Benzyl Isothiocyanate, Breast Cancer, Broccoli, Brussels Sprouts, Cabbage, Cancer, Cancer Stem Cells, Carcinogenesis, Cell Migration, Cruciferous Vegetables, Cyclooxygenase, Diet, Food, Head and Neck Cancer, Head and Neck Cancer, Hematological Cancer, Isothiocyanates, Lung Cancer, Nutrition, Pancreatic Cancer, Phenethyl Isothiocyanate, Proliferation, Prostate Cancer, Sulforaphane, Tumor Initiation, Tumor Progression, Tumor Promotion, Vegetables, Watercress.

INTRODUCTION

Numerous studies have indicated that certain phytochemicals produced by cruciferous vegetables have the capability of being used as both a chemopreventive and chemotherapeutic agent [1-3]. Cruciferous vegetables include broccoli, Indian cress, cabbage, Brussels sprouts, and watercress [4]. Isothiocyanates (ITCs) are the phytochemicals produced by vegetables in the Cruciferae family reported to induce robust anti-cancer effects [2, 5, 6]. ITCs are generated naturally from the hydrolysis of glucosinolates, which are a secondary metabolite found in cruciferous vegetables, and contain a β-D-thioglucose group, a sulfonated oxime moiety, and a variable side chain [7]. A cruciferous vegetable produces ITCs as a defense mechanism when the plant is damaged or "under attack". This family of vegetables spatially separates glucosinolates (cytoplasm) from the defense-related enzyme myrosinase (external surface of the plant cell wall), and when the plant is damaged or chewed the enzyme and glucosinolate are brought into contact, and the glucosinolate undergoes a Lossen rearrangement creating the ITC product [8]. The glucosinolate precursor dictates the type of ITC produced (Table **1**). There are currently over a 100 glucosinolates identified, but not all of the corresponding ITCs appear to have anti-carcinogenic properties [2]. Examination of the literature suggests that the ITCs most frequently investigated for their anti-cancer effects are sulforaphane (SFN), benzyl- (BITC), and phenethyl (PEITC) isothiocyanate, and are therefore the main focus of this chapter (Fig. **1**).

*Address Correspondence to Pier Paolo Claudio: Nutrition and Cancer Center, Department of Biochemistry and Microbiology, Joan C. Edwards School of Medicine, Marshall University, Byrd Biotechnology Science Center, 1700 Third Avenue, Huntington WV, 25755; E-mail: claudiop@marshall.edu

Pier Paolo Claudio and Richard M. Niles (Eds)

Table 1: Isothiocyanates with their corresponding glucosinolate precursor and food source

Isothiocyanate	Glucosinolate (precursor)	Food Sources
Benzyl Isothiocyanate (BITC)	Glucotropaeolin	Cabbage, garden cress, Indian cress
Phenethyl Isothiocyanate (PEITC)	Gluconasturtiin	Watercress
Sulforaphane (SFN)	Glucoraphanin	Broccoli, Brussels sprouts, cabbage

All ITCs, including SFN, BITC, and PEITC have the same R-N=C=S structure. The reactive group is the sulfur containing N=C=S functional group, which is a strong electrophile and can undergo a nucleophilic attack [9]. The N=C=S group is reported to selectively bind to thiol-containing cysteines and ε-amino containing lysine forming thiocarbamates and thioureas, respectively [5]. ITCs are suggested to form thiocarbamates at a 10^3 to 10^4 faster rate than thioureas, but are less stable [5, 9]. The ability of ITCs to target cysteine residues is significant, because cysteine residues are often found in the catalytic site of enzymes [5]. The binding to cysteine residues is suggested to be one way in which ITCs can alter signal transduction and redox status [2].

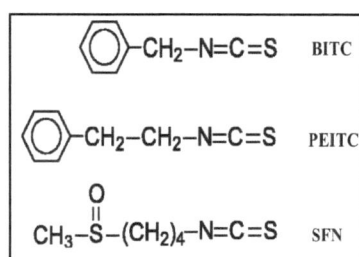

Figure 1: Chemical structure of BITC, PEITC, and SFN.

The R group of ITCs varies significantly, and can be either an alkyl or aryl group. For example, SFN contains an alkyl side chain, where as PEITC and BITC's side chain is an aryl group (Fig. **1**). Proteomics studies have indicated that the R group may play an important role in the targets of ITCs [5, 10]. In A549 cells ^{14}C-SFN was shown to bind to only 16 proteins, whereas ^{14}C-PEITC was shown to target more than 30 proteins [5]. Additionally, a difference in the mechanism of action has been reported when investigating PEITC and SFN's involvement in cell cycle and apoptosis [8, 9]. Furthermore, PEITC and BITC are reported to inhibit cellular proliferation, induce apoptosis, and inhibit cellular migration at significantly lower concentrations compared to SFN [3, 6, 11, 12]. This has also been supported in animal models [2, 7, 13].

Regardless of the mechanism SFN, BITC, and PEITC have all shown to inhibit the growth of many cancerous cell lines, including lung, prostate, and breast [14-18]. However, when considering an effective treatment for any disease one must assesses whether or not the treatment is feasible in humans. Many phytochemicals or polyphenols have indicated promising results in cell culture, but the serum concentrations needed to observe similar effects in humans has not been achieved. The oral bioavailability of ITCs is reported to be high; therefore suggesting that they may be a better treatment option than other phytochemicals. PEITC is described to have a high oral bioavailability in both animals and humans [8]. Additionally, the AUC per os (p.o.) and intravenous (i.v.) administration of PEITC does not appear to differ significantly in mice and rats [8, 19]. Interestingly, increasing the dose of PEITC increases the half-life, and decreases the clearance [2, 7, 8]. ITC metabolites are secreted in the urine and the saturation of the enzymes involved in the metabolism of ITCs may be an explanation for the decreased clearance [7]. The bioavailability of SFN is also described to be high in animals and humans, however there is limited data on the oral bioavailability in humans. In male Wistar rats 82% of SFN has shown to be bioavailable [19]. The half-life and AUC of SFN is lower than that reported of PEITC. PEITC has a half-life of 3.7 to 4.9 hours; whereas the half-life of SFN is only reported to be 1.8 hrs [8]. Bioavailability information, as well as pharmacokinetic information for BITC is currently unavailable. However, accumulation of all ITCs into cells is suggested to be rapid, and the intracellular concentration is reported to be several hundred-fold greater than the extracellular concentration [2]. This observation has been supported in mouse pancreatic endothelial and fibroblast cells, as well as in human prostate and colon cancer cell lines [2, 8]. ITCs have been also reported to reach many tissues because they are coupled to serum albumin and can be systemically transported throughout the body and be released into tissues.

When considering the transition from bench to bedside, bioavailability is critical for the success of ITCs, but methods to determine ITC concentrations in humans are still being fine-tuned. The problem with many of the original methods used for ITC quantification was that they could only determine total ITC concentration and not specific ITC conjugates. Also, the method for determining ITC concentration in the urine *vs.* the blood may need to be different [2, 8]. ITCs are excreted mainly in the urine; therefore, the urine concentration is very high. The concentration in the blood is much lower, and the detection method in the serum needs to be more sensitive to be able to detect the low levels of ITCs [8, 20]. The test also needs to be specific for a certain ITC, not just ITCs in general. Cyclocondensation is a sensitive test to detect ITCs; however, it can only identify the total ITC concentration. This reaction also cannot distinguish between ITCs and other thionyl compounds. When using blood samples, the cyclocondensation reaction is not sufficient enough for ITC quantification. An assay using polyethylene glycol followed by membrane ultrafiltration is suggested to be better for ITC identification in blood [8]. The advantage of this method is that it allows specific ITCs to be identified.

Although, a better understanding of the pharmacokinetic and pharmacodynamics of ITCs is needed, research on ITCs is very promising, and could pave the way for new therapeutic options. Cancer is a multi-stage process involving initiation, promotion and progression. ITCs are suggested to target each of these stages. ITCs are shown to slow cellular growth, induce apoptosis, and inhibit metastasis in cell culture and animal models [1-3, 6]. Additionally, ITCs are also becoming promising adjuvant therapies to both chemo- and radiation therapy [21, 22].

The objective of this chapter is to briefly review the evidence for the benefits SFN, BITC, and/or PEITC treatment in both preventing and treating multiple cancer types, as well as a rational mechanism for these effects. Treatment options for many cancers, especially advanced cancers are still insufficient. Additionally, many current therapies are associated with debilitating side effects and toxicities. Therefore, new and alternative treatment options that are shown to have limited toxicity, such as treatment with ITCs, need to be explored to help push cancer therapy towards a positive direction.

MECHANISM OF ACTION

The mechanism of action involved in the anti-carcinogenic and anti-tumor activity of ITCs has not been fully elucidated. However, the mechanism involved in ITCs ability to inhibit carcinogenesis is more fully understood and involves the inhibition of carcinogen activation. ITCs are known to inhibit the activity of several cytochrome p450s (CYP450), which are Phase I enzymes involved in normal metabolic metabolism, but also carcinogen activation [1, 4, 9]. By inhibiting the activity of CYP450s the ITCs can prevent DNA adduct formation and the subsequent mutation leading to a transformed cell, thereby preventing carcinogenesis. ITCs also induce certain Phase II enzymes, like GST, through activation of the Keap-1/Nrf2 pathway [2, 9]. The induction of Phase II enzymes helps dispose of activated carcinogens by transforming the carcinogen into a water-soluble compound that can be excreted *via* the urine [9]. Additionally, ITCs are shown to rapidly reduce the concentration of GSH in the cell, which can allow ITCs to inhibit progression of cancer. Hyperplasic cells usually have mutations that lead to an increase of reactive oxygen species (ROS). A depletion of GSH is shown induce apoptosis in these various cell lines, because the cells can no longer effectively deal with ROS.

The mechanisms involved in the anti-tumor activity of ITCs are more complex, and include several different molecular pathways (Fig. **2**). Additionally, the type of ITC as well as the concentration appears to have a significant effect on the mechanism of action. ITCs have been described to induce apoptosis and cell cycle arrest, as well target angiogenesis and migration through various mechanisms of action [1, 2]. The multiple signaling cascades targeted by ITCs include the AKT, ERK, and p38 kinase pathways that lead to apoptosis and cell cycle arrest [2, 7, 23, 24]. The mechanism involved in ITCs ability to trigger apoptosis is complex and therefore deserves some discussion. SFN, PEITC, and BITC are all shown to decrease the anti-apoptotic proteins Bcl-2 and Bcl-XL [7, 25]. Additionally, these ITCs induce caspase-3 activity and PARP cleavage [1, 21, 26]. Work on PEITC suggests this ITC has the ability to stimulate caspase-3, -8, and-9 [2]. Although, it was published in leukemia cells that caspase-8 is critical and caspase-3 only provides a supporting role [27]. This suggests that cell apoptosis induced by ITCs works through both the extrinsic and intrinsic mechanism. The pro-apoptotic protein BID also appears to be cleaved in response to ITC treatment indicating that the c-Jun terminal kinase (JNK) pathway is a target of ITCs [7, 28]. SFN, BITC, and PEITC, have all shown to target the JNK pathway in various cancer cells. Interestingly, in OVAR-3 cells, PEITC suppressed the activation of Akt and ERK1/2, but activated the p38 and JNK1/2 pathway.

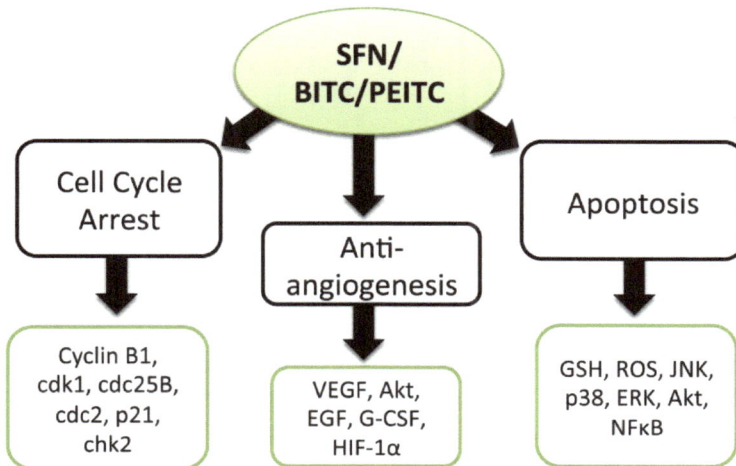

Figure 2: Molecular pathways targeted by SFN, BITC, and PEITC. The antitumor activity of ITCs affects various molecular targets that inhibit cell cycle and angiogenesis, as well as inducing apoptosis.

SFN and PEITC induce apoptosis in numerous cancer cell lines; however, they have different molecular targets. A distinct difference is observed in the induction of apoptosis [7]. PEITC and SFN appear to use different initial signals to trigger apoptosis [5, 7]. The initiation of apoptosis by PEITC is suggested to occur after PEITC binds to tubulin. Dysfunction of tubulin increases the cleavage of caspase-8 and-9. SFN does not appear to have a strong affinity for tubulin, but does induce ROS more potently that PEITC. Other differences are observed between the mechanisms of action involved in the inhibition of cell cycle progression. PEITC, BITC, and SFN all inhibit Chk2 and Cdk1 leading to cell cycle arrest, but only PEITC and BITC are reported to down-regulate cyclin A, D, and E [3, 6, 24, 25, 28, 29].

The mechanism involved in the inhibition of angiogenesis links back to the pathways mentioned to be targeted during the induction of apoptosis. ITCs are known to inhibit the Akt pathway, and this pathway activates mTOR, which consequently activates the 4E-Binding protein (4E-BP). The 4E-BP regulates expression of HIF-1α. SFN, PEITC, and BITC inhibit HIF-1α expression and subsequently factors regulated by HIF-1α that are involved in angiogenesis and epithelial to mesenchymal transition (EMT) [18, 30, 31]. Treatment of prostate cancer PC-3 cells with PEITC also decreased expression of the angiogenic factors, epidermal growth factor, and colony-stimulating factor [23]. PEITC and BITC both cause a decrease in the expression of vascular endothelial growth factor [29]. BITC, SFN, and PEITC have all been shown to inhibit migration of cancer cells [14, 30-33]. BITC and PEITC have also been shown to suppress the metastatic potential of breast and NSCLC cells *in vivo* and *in vitro*. Suppression of metastasis is suggested to occur through modulation of metastasis-related gene expression and inhibition of the Akt/NF-kB pathway. All three ITCs have been demonstrated to inhibit NF-kB activity in a dose dependent manner. The inhibition of NF-kB activity appears to be a critical target of ITCs that can lead to the inhibition of cell growth, induce apoptosis, and inhibit migration.

USES IN CANCER THERAPY

Based on the interactions described in the above section, it is apparent that ITCs could potentially play a significant role in prevention and treatment of various types of cancer. In addition to inhibiting cell growth, inducing apoptosis, and decreasing metastasis, ITCs are also shown to sensitize cancer cells to several chemotherapeutic agents, including cisplatin. ITCs also target cancer stem cell (CSC) populations, which are the major cause for cancer recurrence and drug resistance. According to the "cancer stem cell" theory, tumors are not to be viewed as simple monoclonal expansions of transformed cells, but rather as complex tissues where abnormal growth originates from a pathological minority of cancer stem cells. These cells have maintained stem-like characteristics in that they proliferate very slowly and have an inherent capacity to self-renew and differentiate into phenotypically heterogeneous, aberrant progeny. The following sections give a limited overview of studies that have reported the anti-cancer effects of ITCs in both *in vivo* and *in vitro* model systems.

Lung Cancer

Epidemiological studies indicate that ITC consumption reduces the risk of lung cancer [12]. The nitrosamine, 4-(methylnitrosamino)-1-(3-pyridyl)-1-butanone (NNK), is found in cigarettes and is a major pro-carcinogen linked to lung cancer formation [2]. Several studies have investigated if certain ITCs can inhibit the formation of lung cancer induced by NNK. These studies have led to a Phase II clinical trial (NCT00691132) is investigating the effects of PEITC in participants who smoke only deuterated NNK cigarettes. The objective of this study is to determine if PEITC consumption affects the urinary levels of biomarkers of NNK in current smokers. This research group is studying if there are changes in proliferation, or an increase in apoptotic bodies in lung biopsies taken after ingesting PEITC or placebo [12]. In animal models SFN and PEITC have both shown to inhibit lung tumor formation and progression [2, 12]. SFN and PEITC both induced apoptosis in lung tissues of A/J mice after cigarette carcinogens had induced a lung adenoma. This study implies that these compounds may inhibit the development of adenomas to adenocarcinomas in the lung [12]. In cell culture experiments using various NSCLC cell lines SFN, BITC, and PEITC have all shown to inhibit cellular proliferation at low concentrations [21, 29, 34]. Additionally, both SFN and PEITC induced apoptosis in A549 lung cells after treatment with 20 µM and 40 µM of the each ITC for 24 hrs [34]. In several studies PEITC was shown to be a stronger inducer of apoptosis than SFN. PEITC and BITC were reported to reduce migration and invasion of the highly metastatic NSCLC cell line, L9981 [29]. This study also demonstrated that BITC and PEITC inhibited phosphorylated AKT, while also inhibiting activity of NF-kB and reducing metastasis related gene expression [29]. One of the first reports of chemosensitization in response to ITC treatment was also reported in NSCLC [21]. Pasqua *et al.* (2010) showed that pretreatment with 10 µM of BITC or PEITC sensitized NCI-H596 cells to cisplatin.

Breast Cancer

ITC consumption, in general, has been linked with a reduction in risk of breast cancer and is now being investigated as a breast cancer treatment option [4, 18, 35]. Currently, there are three clinical trials recruiting breast cancer patients, all of which are in Phase II. Two studies are investigating if the consumption of broccoli sprout extract (SFN) can alter proliferation of breast tissue (NCT00982319 and NCT00843167). The study being completed by the Shannon lab in Oregon (NCT00843167) is focusing on HDAC activity (acetylated histone expression) and apoptosis in women diagnosed with breast cancer, ductal carcinoma *in situ* and/or atypical hyperplasia. Additionally, a clinical trial being sponsored by the Sidney Kimmel Comprehensive Cancer Center is looking at the protective effects of topical SFN on radiation-induced dermatitis in women undergoing external-beam radiation therapy for breast cancer. Furthermore, several animal feeding studies have indicated that ITC treatment can inhibit breast cancer carcinogenesis, and recently it was published that BITC consumption could inhibit mammary carcinogenesis in MMTV-neu mice. This study suggested that a diet supplemented with 3mmol BITC/kg of chow could significantly decrease the number of Ki-67 positive cells, and increase the number of apoptotic bodies in mammary tumors [35]. SFN, BITC, and PEITC have also shown to inhibit cell growth and induce apoptosis in breast cancer cell lines, such as the MCF-7 cell line [6, 34]. Additionally, BITC was reported to inhibit epithelial-mesenchymal transition (EMT) in the MDA-MB-231 human breast cancer cell line. This was also supported in xenografted human breast cancer cells [36]. Moreover, BITC was shown to inhibit hypoxia inducible factor (HIF1-α) expression and activity in MCF-7 cells by targeting the 4E binding protein 1 (4E-BP1) [16, 18]. Studies that target cancer stem cells are currently of great interest, and SFN was found to decrease aldehyde dehydrogenase-1 (ALDH-1) positive cells in the MCF-7 and SUM159 human breast cancer cell lines [37]. ALDH-1 is a known cancer stem cell marker in breast cancer. Additionally, daily injection of SFN (50 mg/kg) for 2 weeks reduced the number of ALDH-1 positive cells by 50% in non-obese/severe combined immunodeficient mice with SUM159 xenograft tumors. Treatment with SFN also decreases the number of primary mammospheres which are known to have cancer stem-like cell properties, by 8- to 125-fold in these two cell lines [37].

Prostate Cancer

Epidemiological evidence is mixed when investigating the relationship between cruciferous vegetable consumption and prostate cancer. In eight case-control studies published since 1990, four studies have shown a significantly lower incidence of prostate cancer in men who consumed large amounts of cruciferous vegetable [1, 4, 17]. The other four studies indicated that there was no significant difference. Limiting the analysis to men who are positive for prostate specific antigen (PSA) appears to decrease some bias and show a stronger link between ITCs and the reduction of prostate cancer [17]. A curret clinical trial (NCT01265953) is attempting to identify mechanisms by which SFN capsules can alter gene expression *via* epigenetic modifications in patients at risk for prostate cancer development. This study is particularly interested in studying SFN's effects on HDAC and DNA methylation on biopsies from men at risk for prostate cancer. In addition to the clinical trials, much work *in vivo* and *in vitro* has been done investigating ITCs ability to both inhibit and target prostate cancer [1, 15, 23, 28]. ITCs are also shown to target prostate tumors, and there is a Phase II clinical trial (NCT01228084) which recruiting patients with recurrent prostate cancer. This trial is investigating if treatment with SFN can decrease PSA levels within 20 weeks of the SFN treatment. Xiao *et al.* (2010) recently published that PEITC can sensitize PC-3 and DU145 cells to docetaxel [38]. In the same study, intraperitoneally injected PEITC in combination with docetaxel was shown to upregulate pro-apoptotic proteins (Bax and Bak) greater than compared with PEITC or docetaxel treatment alone in PC-3 xenografts in male athymic mice [38]. Additionally, treatment with PEITC and docetaxel inhibited average tumor volume significantly more than either treatment alone. One mechanism proposed by which ITCs can exhibit antitumor effects on prostate cancer cells is *via* the JAK/STAT3/IL6 pathway [15, 28, 39]. Two independent studies have suggested that both SFN and PEITC can inhibit STAT3 activation and IL-6 production. Inhibition of STAT3 activation is proposed to be one way in which ITCs produce pro-apoptotic effects [15]. Additionally, BITC treatment was found to inhibit cellular growth and to induce G2/M cell cycle arrest in DU145 cells [28]. Treatment with BITC also stimulated apoptosis in DU145 cells through the release of AIF and Endo G from the mitochondria, and also promoted caspase-3 activation [40].

Pancreatic Cancer

Currently, there are no clinical trials investigating the effects of ITCs on the prevention or treatment of pancreatic cancer. However, several animal models have suggested that BITC, PEITC, and SFN can inhibit pancreatic tumor formation. For example, in an animal model using Syrian Hamsters PEITC was shown to inhibit the formation of N-nitrobis (2-oxypropyl) amine (BOP)-induced pancreatic tumors [41]. In cell culture BITC and PEITC have been shown to inhibit NF-kB activity, STAT3 activation, and induce reactive oxygen species [24, 42, 43]. Additionally, SFN alone or in combination with TRAIL (tumor necrosis factor-related apoptosis-inducing ligand) was shown to significantly reduce the growth of pancreatic tumors that are rich in tumor initiating cells, or cancer stem cells, while not causing cytotoxic or adverse effects in normal pancreatic cancer cells [44]. Rausch *et al.* (2010) also suggested that SFN in combination with sorafenib has a synergistic effect in targeting pancreatic cancer stem cells, by decreasing clonogenicity, spheroid formation, and ALDH1 activity [45].

Hematological Cancer

Literature is indicating that PEITC has been of significant interest in treating various hematological cancers, such as leukemia, Acute Myeloid Leukemia (AML), and multiple myeloma [2]. A Phase I clinical trial (NCT00968461) is scheduled to begin in January of 2012 by the MD Anderson Cancer Center. The objective of the study is to identify the highest tolerable dose of orally administered PEITC that can be given to patients who have lymphoproliferative disorders and have previously been treated with the drug fludarabine. Of great clinical interest is a study which demonstrated that primary Chronic Lymphocytic Leukemia (CLL) cells, both resistant and responsive to fludarabine, were highly sensitive to PEITC with an IC_{50} of 5.4 and 5.1 µmol/L, respectively [27]. However, normal lymphocytes did no show sensitivity to the same level of PEITC until 27 µmol/L [27]. In other cell culture experiments, PEITC has demonstrated to inhibit cellular growth and induce apoptosis in the U937, Jurkat, and HL-60 human leukemia cell lines [46]. SFN and PEITC have been shown to inhibit proliferation of primary human acute myeloid leukemia (AML) cells *in vivo* and *in vitro* [46, 47]. In AML cell lines SFN and PEITC both induced cleavage of PARP and caspases-3 and-9 in a concentration dependent manner [3, 48]. PEITC has also been shown to inhibit NF-kB, activate the JNK pathway, and inhibit the AKT pathway in the U937 human leukemia cell line, indicating a mechanism through which PEITC can induce apoptosis [46].

Head and Neck Cancer

Studies investigating the effects of ITCs on Head and Neck Cancer are limited. A few epidemiologic and basic research studies have suggested that a diet rich in cruciferous vegetables may reduce the risk of developing primary head and neck tumors [49]. As with NSCLC, smoking is the biggest risk factor for head and neck squamous cell carcinoma (HNSCC) [50]. Numerous reports using both animal models and human subjects suggest that ITCs can reduce the activity of carcinogens found in cigarettes, such as NNK [41]. All the *in vivo* studies to date looked at inhibition of lung carcinogenesis in response to cigarette carcinogens. Future studies need to investigate if ITCs can reduce the incidence of NNK induced HNSCC carcinogenesis in animal models. However, as with the other cancers described BITC, PEITC and SFN inhibit proliferation *in vitro* of HNSCC cell lines [2, 49]. BITC induces caspase-3 and PARP cleavage in the UM-22B and 1483 HNSCC cell lines in a time dependent manner [51]. In addition, BITC induces rapid activation of p38 MAPK, as well as activation of p44/MAPK in these same cell lines [49, 51]. Another HNSCC study showed that a combination of SFN and radiation might produce a synergistic effect in decreasing proliferation in four HNSCC cell lines [22]. This study also indicated that a combination of SFN and chemotherapy increased apoptosis of HNSCC cell lines greater than treatment with either SFN or radiation alone. Data generated in our laboratory also suggest that BITC can chemosensitize the highly resistant HN12 and HN30 HNSCC cell lines to cisplatin. Additionally, we observed that BITC appears to inhibit migration of the HN12 HNSCC cell line in a dose dependent manner (Fig. 3).

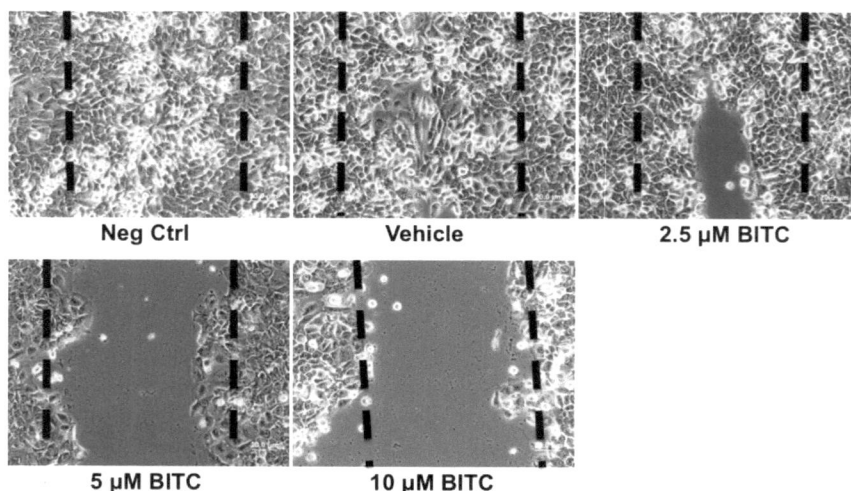

Figure 3: BITC decreases migration of HN12 cells in a wound-healing assay after 24 hrs. HN12 cells were seeded in 6-well dishes and grown to 90% confluency. Cells were then placed in low serum (0.5%) media overnight, before scratches were made. Cells were treated with 2.5, 5, or 10 µM BITC for 1 hour. Images were taken before treatment and after 24 hrs. Dotted lines represent the scratch size at time 0. Vehicle was DMSO. Representative Images at magnification 100X.

CONCLUSIONS

Although the results from clinical trials are limited for ITCs, literature suggests that both SFN and PEITC are safe treatment options that can reach clinically relevant concentrations. ITCs are a very unique treatment, in that they appear to prevent and treat cancer. The ability of SFN, PEITC, and BITC to inhibit cellular proliferation, to induce apoptosis, and to inhibit angiogenesis in cancer cells has been extensively studied. Additionally, studies *in vivo* and *in vitro* suggest that certain ITCs may chemosensitize cancer cells. Interestingly, ITCs target the tumor initiating or cancer stem cells population in breast, prostate, and pancreatic cancer. Furthermore, ITCs inhibit metastasis both *in vitro* and *in vivo*. The mechanisms of action for ITCs are complex and work through multiple pathways. The ability of ITCs to bind to a diverse array of proteins indicates that additional mechanisms through which ITCs exhibit their effects are yet to be identified. A more complete understanding of the effects of these ITCs are needed, as well as a better understanding of their safety, which will help progress ITCs into future therapeutic options.

REFERENCES

[1]   Clarke JD, Dashwood RH, Ho E. Multi-targeted prevention of cancer by sulforaphane. Cancer Lett 2008; 269(2): 291-304.

[2]   Wu X, Zhou QH, Xu K. Are isothiocyanates potential anti-cancer drugs? ActaPharmacol Sin 2009; 30(5): 501-12.

[3]   Zhang Y, Tang L, Gonzalez V. Selected isothiocyanates rapidly induce growth inhibition of cancer cells. Mol Cancer Ther 2003; 2(10): 1045-52.

[4]   Kelloff GJ, Crowell JA, Steele VE, *et al.* Progress in cancer chemoprevention. Ann N Y AcadSci 1999; 889: 1-13.

[5]   Mi L, Hood BL, Stewart NA, *et al.* Identification of potential protein targets of isothiocyanates by proteomics. Chem Res Toxicol 2011; 24(10): 1735-43.

[6]   Zhang Y. Molecular mechanism of rapid cellular accumulation of anticarcinogenicisothiocyanates. Carcinogenesis 2001; 22(3): 425-31.

[7]   Cheung KL, Kong AN. Molecular targets of dietary phenethyl isothiocyanate and sulforaphane for cancer chemoprevention. Aaps J 2009; 12(1): 87-97.

[8]   Lamy E, Scholtes C, Herz C, Mersch-Sundermann V. Pharmacokinetics and pharmacodynamics of isothiocyanates. Drug Metab Rev 2011; 43(3): 387-407.

[9]   Nakamura Y, Miyoshi N. Electrophiles in foods: the current status of isothiocyanates and their chemical biology. BiosciBiotechnolBiochem 2010; 74(2): 242-55.

[10]   Mi L, Xiao Z, Veenstra TD, Chung FL. Proteomic identification of binding targets of isothiocyanates: A perspective on techniques. J Proteomics 2011; 74(7): 1036-44.

[11]   Cavell BE, Syed Alwi SS, Donlevy A, Packham G. Anti-angiogenic effects of dietary isothiocyanates: mechanisms of action and implications for human health. BiochemPharmacol 2011; 81(3): 327-36.

[12]   Conaway CC, Wang CX, Pittman B, *et al.* Phenethyl isothiocyanate and sulforaphane and their N-acetylcysteine conjugates inhibit malignant progression of lung adenomas induced by tobacco carcinogens in A/J mice. Cancer Res 2005; 65(18): 8548-57.

[13]   Mi L, Wang X, Govind S, *et al.* The role of protein binding in induction of apoptosis by phenethyl isothiocyanate and sulforaphane in human non-small lung cancer cells. Cancer Res 2007; 67(13): 6409-16.

[14]   Boreddy SR, Sahu RP, Srivastava SK. Benzyl isothiocyanate suppresses pancreatic tumor angiogenesis and invasion by inhibiting HIF-alpha/VEGF/Rho-GTPases: pivotal role of STAT-3. PLoS One 2011; 6(10): e25799.

[15]   Gong A, He M, Krishna Vanaja D, *et al.* Phenethyl isothiocyanate inhibits STAT3 activation in prostate cancer cells. MolNutr Food Res 2009; 53(7): 878-86.

[16]   Hunakova L, Sedlakova O, Cholujova D, *et al.* Modulation of markers associated with aggressive phenotype in MDA-MB-231 breast carcinoma cells by sulforaphane. Neoplasma 2009; 56(6): 548-56.

[17]   Shukla S, Gupta S. Dietary agents in the chemoprevention of prostate cancer. Nutr Cancer 2005; 53(1): 18-32.

[18]   Syed Alwi SS, Cavell BE, Telang U, *et al.* In vivo modulation of 4E binding protein 1 (4E-BP1) phosphorylation by watercress: a pilot study. Br J Nutr 2010; 104(9): 1288-96.

[19]   Ji Y, Kuo Y, Morris ME. Pharmacokinetics of dietary phenethyl isothiocyanate in rats. Pharm Res 2005; 22(10): 1658-66.

[20]   Steck SE, Gammon MD, Hebert JR, Wall DE, Zeisel SH. GSTM1, GSTT1, GSTP1, and GSTA1 polymorphisms and urinary isothiocyanate metabolites following broccoli consumption in humans. J Nutr 2007; 137(4): 904-9.

[21]   Di Pasqua AJ, Hong C, Wu MY, *et al.* Sensitization of non-small cell lung cancer cells to cisplatin by naturally

occurring isothiocyanates. Chem Res Toxicol 2010; 23(8): 1307-9.

[22] Kotowski U, Heiduschka G, Brunner M, *et al*. Radiosensitization of head and neck cancer cells by the phytochemical agent sulforaphane. StrahlentherOnkol 2011; 187(9): 575-80.

[23] Kim JH, Xu C, Keum YS, *et al*. Inhibition of EGFR signaling in human prostate cancer PC-3 cells by combination treatment with beta-phenylethyl isothiocyanate and curcumin. Carcinogenesis 2006; 27(3): 475-82.

[24] Zhang R, Loganathan S, Humphreys I, Srivastava SK. Benzyl isothiocyanate-induced DNA damage causes G2/M cell cycle arrest and apoptosis in human pancreatic cancer cells. J Nutr 2006; 136(11): 2728-34.

[25] Chen YR, Han J, Kori R, Kong AN, Tan TH. Phenylethyl isothiocyanate induces apoptotic signaling via suppressing phosphatase activity against c-Jun N-terminal kinase. J BiolChem 2002; 277(42): 39334-42.

[26] Cheung KL, Khor TO, Yu S, Kong AN. PEITC induces G1 cell cycle arrest on HT-29 cells through the activation of p38 MAPK signaling pathway. Aaps J 2008; 10(2): 277-81.

[27] Trachootham D, Zhang H, Zhang W, *et al*. Effective elimination of fludarabine-resistant CLL cells by PEITC through a redox-mediated mechanism. Blood 2008; 112(5): 1912-22.

[28] Xu C, Shen G, Yuan X, *et al*. ERK and JNK signaling pathways are involved in the regulation of activator protein 1 and cell death elicited by three isothiocyanates in human prostate cancer PC-3 cells. Carcinogenesis 2006; 27(3): 437-45.

[29] Wu X, Zhu Y, Yan H, *et al*. Isothiocyanates induce oxidative stress and suppress the metastasis potential of humannon-small cell lung cancer cells. BMC Cancer 2010; 10: 269.

[30] Wang XH, Cavell BE, Syed Alwi SS, Packham G. Inhibition of hypoxia inducible factor by phenethylisothiocyanate. BiochemPharmacol 2009; 78(3): 261-72.

[31] Xiao D, Singh SV. Phenethyl isothiocyanate inhibits angiogenesis *in vitro* and *ex vivo*. Cancer Res 2007; 67(5):2239-46.

[32] Asakage M, Tsuno NH, Kitayama J, *et al*. Sulforaphane induces inhibition of human umbilical vein endothelial cellsproliferation by apoptosis. Angiogenesis 2006; 9(2): 83-91.

[33] Prawan A, Saw CL, Khor TO, *et al*. Anti-NF-kappaB and anti-inflammatory activities of synthetic isothiocyanates:effect of chemical structures and cellular signaling. ChemBiol Interact 2009; 179(2-3): 202-11.

[34] Nakamura Y. Chemoprevention by isothiocyanates: molecular basis of apoptosis induction. Forum Nutr 2009; 61:170-81.

[35] Warin R, Chambers WH, Potter DM, Singh SV. Prevention of mammary carcinogenesis in MMTV-neu mice bycruciferous vegetable constituent benzyl isothiocyanate. Cancer Res 2009; 69(24): 9473-80.

[36] Sehrawat A, Singh SV. Benzyl isothiocyanate inhibits epithelial-mesenchymal transition in cultured and xenograftedhuman breast cancer cells. Cancer Prev Res (Phila) 2011; 4(7): 1107-17.

[37] Li Y, Zhang T, Korkaya H, *et al*. Sulforaphane, a dietary component of broccoli/broccoli sprouts, inhibits breastcancer stem cells. Clin Cancer Res 2010; 16(9): 2580-90.

[38] Xiao D, Singh SV. Phenethyl isothiocyanate sensitizes androgen-independent human prostate cancer cells todocetaxel-induced apoptosis *in vitro* and *in vivo*. Pharm Res 2010; 27(4): 722-31.

[39] Xu C, Shen G, Chen C, Gelinas C, Kong AN. Suppression of NF-kappaB and NF-kappaB-regulated gene expressionby sulforaphane and PEITC through IkappaBalpha, IKK pathway in human prostate cancer PC-3 cells. Oncogene2005; 24(28): 4486-95.

[40] Liu KC, Huang YT, Wu PP, *et al*. The roles of AIF and Endo G in the apoptotic effects of benzyl isothiocyanate onDU 145 human prostate cancer cells *via* the mitochondrial signaling pathway. Int J Oncol 2010; 38(3): 787-96.

[41] Nishikawa A, Furukawa F, Uneyama C, *et al*. Chemopreventive effects of phenethyl isothiocyanate on lung andpancreatic tumorigenesis in N-nitrosobis(2-oxopropyl)amine-treated hamsters. Carcinogenesis 1996; 17(6): 1381-4.

[42] Sahu RP, Srivastava SK. The role of STAT-3 in the induction of apoptosis in pancreatic cancer cells by benzylisothiocyanate. J Natl Cancer Inst 2009; 101(3): 176-93.

[43] Basu A, Haldar S. Dietary isothiocyanate mediated apoptosis of human cancer cells is associated with Bcl-xLphosphorylation. Int J Oncol 2008; 33(4): 657-63.

[44] Kallifatidis G, Rausch V, Baumann B, *et al*. Sulforaphane targets pancreatic tumour-initiating cells by NF-kappaBinducedantiapoptoticsignalling. Gut 2009; 58(7): 949-63.

[45] Rausch V, Liu L, Kallifatidis G, *et al*. Synergistic activity of sorafenib and sulforaphane abolishes pancreatic cancerstem cell characteristics. Cancer Res 2010; 70(12): 5004-13.

[46] Gao N, Budhraja A, Cheng S, *et al*. Phenethyl isothiocyanate exhibits antileukemic activity *in vitro* and *in vivo* byinactivation of Akt and activation of JNK pathways. Cell Death Dis 2011; 2: e140.

[47] Gao SS, Chen XY, Zhu RZ, Choi BM, Kim BR. Sulforaphane induces glutathione S-transferaseisozymes whichdetoxify aflatoxin B(1)-8,9-epoxide in AML 12 cells. Biofactors 2010; 36(4): 289-96.

[48] Xu K, Thornalley PJ. Studies on the mechanism of the inhibition of human leukaemia cell growth by

dietaryisothiocyanates and their cysteine adducts *in vitro*. BiochemPharmacol 2000; 60(2): 221-31.

[49]   Fowke JH. Head and neck cancer: a case for inhibition by isothiocyanates and indoles from cruciferous vegetables.Eur J Cancer Prev 2007; 16(4): 348-56.

[50]   Wrangle JM, Khuri FR. Chemoprevention of squamous cell carcinoma of the head and neck. CurrOpinOncol 2007;19(3): 180-7.

[51]   Lui VW, Wentzel AL, Xiao D, *et al*. Requirement of a carbon spacer in benzyl isothiocyanate-mediated cytotoxicityand MAPK activation in head and neck squamous cell carcinoma. Carcinogenesis 2003; 24(10): 1705-12.

Index

www.ingramcontent.com/pod-product-compliance
Lightning Source LLC
Chambersburg PA
CBHW041719210326
41598CB00007B/705